CONFESSIONS OF A STARCHIVORE

CONFESSIONS OF
A STARCHIVORE

Lose Weight Gain Health Eating Carbs

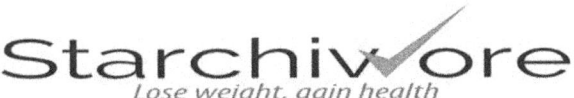
Lose weight, gain health

www.ImaStarchivore.com

**Eat *carbs*, lose weight, feel great!
It's *not* your fault! It's the *food*!**

Christopher Carnrick

ISBN: 1508953805
ISBN 13: 9781508953807

Table of Contents

Mil Gracias (A Thousand Thanks) To

Dr. John McDougall, who has dedicated his career to spreading the word that a starch-centered diet creates health and weight loss. He took information from those who mentored him and forged ahead. As much as I didn't want to agree with this way of eating, the results were direct proof that it works!

Mary McDougall, first of all, rode the wild ride with John in the journey. If it was not for Mary's work in the kitchen working with starch-centered food, I doubt this plan would be livable. Together as a team, they made a huge impact. On a personal note, I can say that you won't meet a nicer couple, either!

Personal Trainer Francisco Javier González Montilla, who went above and beyond his call of duty to help me achieve success. His encouragement and enthusiasm pushed me when I thought I could not do more. I had low points, and he encouraged me through them, and he celebrated the high points. He is truly a gifted trainer.

Arthur Scott Knighton, who joined me on this venture at first in the spirit of solidarity and later because of the major positive health changes in his own life. I could not have had this adventure without my chico. Thank you so much!

Photographer Maria Lopez, Vélez-Málaga, España, for making me comfortable taking my shirt off in front of a camera!

Heather McDougall who is the most amazing coordinator, and the most patient and sweetest human I have ever met! The ten-day live-in program in Santa Rosa was life changing.

Also thank you for the inspiration and motivation: Jeff Novick, Rip Esselstyn, Dr. Caldwell Esselstyn, T. Colin Campbell, and Brendan Brazier.

A starchivore is an animal anatomically and physiologically adapted to mainly eating starch and plant material—for example potatoes, rice, corn, and beans—for the main component of its diet.

Warning: This book will challenge what many of us have accepted to be absolutes in life regarding our food. I know because I was one who scoffed and searched for any research that would counter this way of eating. It was after a long journey when I finally discovered the true silver bullet, without fads, without surgery, without hunger, and without pain.

Just imagine for a moment sitting down to a nice big bowl of mashed potatoes with gravy and a salad. Now imagine going back for seconds, then thirds. Now try, if you can, to imagine doing all this without guilt and with the knowledge that you are losing weight and gaining health.

I am not a physician, nor do I make any claims to be an authority. This book is to share with you how a former fatty—F^2—finally found the key that unlocked the mystery of why I was fat, unhealthy, and in pain.

Many diet plans state, "Results not typical." The information and journey I will share *are* typical, and you can expect the same results that thousands have achieved. The results *are* typical.

Although this educational opportunity provided by Christopher Carnrick may contain materials from Dr. John McDougall, his books and website, the classes and their content are presented entirely independent of the McDougall Program. The use of "McDougall" materials in any form is not an endorsement of the classes being presented, nor should you expect the same weight loss and medical benefits experienced during the ten-day live-in McDougall program (www.drmcdougall.com). Check with your healthcare provider before changing your diet or medications.

What made you decide to read this?

It isn't your fault…it's the food!

If you are reading this, you could possibly have the same feelings and journey that I did. Maybe you have a friend or family member who struggles with weight. My goal is to share my pain with others and possibly be a resource for parents of a child who is struggling with weight issues. Please be warned that I plan to be brutally honest and provide all facts. If you are one of those who is the subject of ridicule because of your weight, I want to let you know it *can* get better. Today I have absolutely no hard feelings toward any of those who taunted me or caused me pain.

First, and most important, you need to know that it really isn't your fault. Yes, we all know that we can make better choices, but some of us are hard-wired to make choices that can cause us to gain weight. It isn't your genes, it isn't your blood type, it isn't a trauma. It is the food!

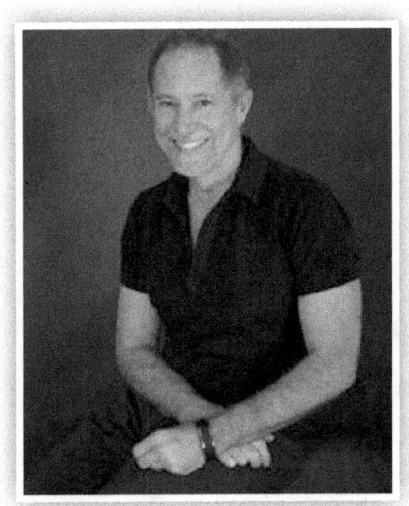

My name is Christopher Carnrick. I am a certified Starch Solution counselor/trainer. I was the owner of two restaurants in Seattle, Washington: Mame's Cabaret and Speedy Gonzales. I am the founder of Casa Cebadillas, in Torrox Pueblo, Spain, which provided themed dinner parties as well as a culinary school. I am also author of the book *Kitchen Disasters: Solutions and Substitutions* and coauthor of *Dinner for Six at 8:00*, and I'm a regular TV personality on a variety of cooking shows on CBS, NBC, and FOX networks.

I love food and creating a festive atmosphere for friends and guests. I was one of those chefs about whom people said, "You can tell he knows good food. Look at his belly."

Today, at almost sixty years old, I am a former fatty—F²— and currently a starchivore. I lost seventy pounds, stopped taking medications, and became healthy, eating all the way, including when I changed my environment to Spain, with all the wine and food. I wanted to share this adventure with you in the hopes that you too can find the success I did. You see, it isn't your fault. It is the food.

So how I did I become a starchivore and why? Read on! Share my journey.

My History

I was not abused and did not have any trauma or anything exotic happen to me—nothing I can point to and place blame for my being fat. I will share that not a day goes by that the first thing I think about when I wake—and the last thing before I go to bed—is my weight. I also worry that all this progress is going to vanish, and one morning I will wake up fat again. I have created for myself all kinds of rules and methods of weighing to manipulate the scale and results. I place it in a particular corner, on a particular crack, press on the counter, and release slowly, being careful not to move. I drink a glass of wine before bed and I am sure to void completely before approaching the scale. I weigh myself before eating anything.

My father was a medical doctor, and my mother a housewife. Family meals were always, in my opinion, wonderful. My mother was a gourmet, and she could make the most incredible dishes. My palate for excellent food was well established. I did, however, yearn for some of the food my friends had to eat, like casseroles. I remember stating once, "Steak, baked potato, and salad, steak, baked potato, and salad! Why can't we have a casserole?" When we did have a casserole, it was creamed tuna with sherry on buttered noodles.

I also remember kids at school telling me how much they hated lima beans. We ate them all the time, and I loved them. Of course, they were cooked by sautéing in butter with onion and a carton of sour cream folded in. Broccoli, another favorite, was served with cauliflower and homemade hollandaise, a rich cheese sauce. See, I was eating vegetables! I couldn't really taste these vegetables because they were covered in fatty sauces. We consumed salads often but usually with avocado and bacon and blue cheese dressing or another mayonnaise-based dressing. Fish, with a browned butter sauce, we ate with scalloped potatoes with cheddar cream sauce and bacon. Weekends and summers at the lake meant grilled chicken, burgers, hot dogs with all the trimmings. These were considered well-balanced meals by most of America.

My first realization of my weight was when I was eight years old. I remember going that summer to a department store in a small town in Texas to buy jeans, preparing for going back to school. I still remember the numbers. My shirt went from a kid's size 16 to an 18, and then I was directed to the young adult section. I didn't understand exactly why I felt ashamed, but there was something in the air. The salesclerk looked down at me with her glassed propped on her nose, fastened around her neck with a cheap chain, and she shook her head and sighed. "No, sir, these ain't gonna fit." Then she said the phrase I learned to loathe. "We are going to have to go to a husky." Husky was a politically correct term for "fatso." Now, with bags of fatso clothes, I was prepared for the new school year. My mother didn't really say anything, but I could see the disappointment in her face after they used the "husky" word.

Going to school as a fat kid is not easy. It is a daily death march. I recently confessed to my mother some of the things that happened to me as a child, and she was appalled and angry that I had not told her. You see, it is a double-edged sword. If I had told her and she'd marched to the school, I would have been labeled for life as the FAT tattletale. I also never shared because it was humiliating, and I didn't want my family to know.

Children can be cruel. I think they focus attention on others to prevent any focus on their own insecurities. A fat kid is an easy target. I was called everything you can imagine. "Fatty,

fatty, two by four, can't get through the bathroom door. Hey, your parents named you Chris, but it is really Crisco. You are all fat! Ha-ha-ha-ha. Hey, I bet you're scared at Thanksgiving, Butterball turkey!"

I began to get sick a great deal, unable to go to school. I can tell you today that the reality was that I was not sick. I developed techniques to avoid school. I knew how I could get away with certain symptoms but not abuse them. When my temperature was taken, if they left the room, I would rub the thermometer between my hands to warm it to the point of one hundred degrees and quickly place back in my mouth. Another technique was to drink very hot water, hold it in my mouth, and swallow right before the thermometer was inserted. I would sneak into the kitchen and grab food. I'd hide it in my pajamas, take it into the bathroom, chew, and then spit it into the toilet, making retching noises. It guaranteed me a day away from school. This was my favorite technique, because around two o'clock in the afternoon, I could declare that I felt much better and have a huge meal.

The illness ploy eventually landed me at my father's office for a fluoroscope to see if I had ulcers. Of course this came out negative. My father was getting suspicious, my mother worried, and my grades were awful! I went from being a good student to a failing student.

If you have siblings, you might be "fat shamed" as well. I was the youngest, and they said I was fat because I was the baby. My oldest sibling was fond of calling me "lard ass." My father was a physician, and in many ways, my being fat was a reflection on his skills as a physician. He would lecture me about calories and portions. He watched me like a hawk as I ate dinner and applauded me when I turned down dessert. Going out for dinner with my father was a fat lesson, as each item requested was scrutinized.

My weight increased, and I remember developing "chub rub." For those of you who never have been fat, let me explain. As your thighs increase in size, they begin rubbing against each other. If you are wearing shorts, the skin will rub together and cause raw spots that are very painful. In school, I remember sitting in class and hearing someone exclaim, "Carnrick has a fat biscuit." *What is a fat biscuit?* you may ask. Let me explain. When your pants rub together so much in the thighs, you begin to rub the material away, eventually making a hole on the inside seam of the pants. The fat presses against the hole and bulges out and looks like a biscuit. I had several pairs of pants with these holes, which I tried to camouflage by adding masking tape or other things to cover the holes. I never shared with my parents that there were worn places in my pants because of the deep humiliation I felt. Inside, I was telling myself that I could have prevented all this by having more self-control and not eating so much.

My mom was more understanding, and she decided to help me and put me on a diet. This was my first of *many* diets I would try. I would start my day drinking a Sego or Metrecal meal replacement drink for breakfast. I would walk home for lunch, and she would get a can of Sego, double chocolate fudge, freeze it, and put it in the blender with Tab diet soda to make a frosty drink for me, and then dinner was a sensible (aka small) meal.

The diet worked. I was losing weight, and my clothes were more comfortable. Then I was rewarded with "treat days." Yes! This meant that after the week of dieting, on the weekend I could eat all I wanted. I devoured food as if I had been starving on an island, and in my mind I justified each bite, saying, "Hey, I deserve this." This was a habit that I continued into my adult life.

Now that I was keenly aware that I was obese, the shame was internalized. I felt there was something wrong with me because I was seriously *hungry*. I would love to say that it was to drown emotions, but the truth is that I was physically hungry. I began to be a secret eater.

The first time I was caught hiding food was the most memorable. When I would walk to my bedroom, I always passed a bookshelf near the kitchen and take a book to read before bed. I would sneak into the kitchen and make a sandwich with anything I could find. This memorable night, it was a macaroni sandwich. I placed the sandwich in the book, placed the book under my arm and walked calmly to my bedroom, only to get stopped by my mother. She noticed something was in the book and took it for inspection. The look of horror on her face flooded me with shame. I was severely scolded, not only for sneaking food but for defacing a book. I went to bed ashamed and with the knowledge that there was something seriously wrong with me.

As I moved on to middle school, the problems continued. I didn't play sports; however, I was required to participate. A sports captain had to pick teams for sports in school. This was a way that everyone, especially me, knew where we stood regarding popularity and physical abilities. One by one, the most athletic and popular were chosen. I was always the "consolation prize." They would rather pick a girl in an iron lung to be on their team than me. You could see the team's look of disappointment when I was assigned to their team.

I grew tired of always being the tackle because I was fat. It was just assumed that maybe if I just stood there, no one could budge me. No one really wanted me on their team now. They just had to figure out how to use this useless piece of flesh that was assigned to them.

One day the coach announced that we were going to wrestle. I had never wrestled in my life, and all I knew about this sport was what I had seen on TV on *Wide World of Wrestling*.

I was teamed with another fat guy, and we were first to have a round. I was panicking because I had no idea what to do. The coach blew the whistle, and immediately I ran toward my opponent, jumped in the air, and performed a body slam. The room roared! I thought, *Hey, maybe I am good at some kind of sport after all.* My opponent down, I ran and leaped in the air and body slammed down again. Everyone was laughing, even my opponent. The coach had tears streaming down his face. They finally pulled me off him and asked if I had ever wrestled before. I said, "No. Am I any good?" Again, howls of laughter filled the room, and they all assured me that what I had done had nothing to do with wrestling.

Even during traumatic times in one's life, young people can be cruel. I was with my parents on our sailboat, headed for Spain, when we were caught in a storm and crashed. My father almost lost his life. It was televised on national TV. When I returned to school, the kids were all laughing. "Of course you survived, Crisco! Fat floats."

So far in this book I have shared some of the ugly parts of being fat. Yes, other kids and adults can be cruel. Society has a standard and norm that I didn't fit. I was fat and deaf, and I had no friends. I lost my hearing in the third grade due to measles, so this just added to the mix. Deaf *and* fat.

Now I want to share how all this can affect a child like me. All the messages you receive—you're strange, you don't fit in, you have nothing to contribute, you're lazy, you wear husky clothes, you're ugly, and so on—can be more dangerous than poor health from obesity. Meaning that as a young kid I considered, thought about, and planned suicide. This is not something I have shared, but I am doing so today because I want every person who struggles with weight to know that they are not alone. It isn't their fault. They are not lazy. They are not unloved. Most important, there is an easy solution that I am going to share later on in this book. I will help you, I will walk with you, I will support you. Hang in there.

As an adult, I was still struggling with weight. I always kept three sets of clothes: thin clothes, fat clothes, and a set I referred to as my "Oh my Gawd, what have I done?" clothes. I weighed every day. Each day I would get on the scale, and the numbers would determine how my day and self-worth would be gauged. I sighed in relief when my weight was the same, celebrate any loss with a food treat, and eat away! I would be miserable if I had gained, feeling that nothing looked good that I wore and that people saw me as fat and lazy. I tried to justify it by declaring it was my genes, and the self-talk would beat me down into a suicidal depression.

I got a job teaching acting at a modeling school in Seattle and was promoted to agency director. Of course, I had to be slender to keep this job. Here I learned all the unhealthy ways to lose weight. Laxative abuse, smoking, starvation, and the one thing I used: swallowing wet cotton balls to feel full. I lost lots of weight. Finally I had a very good friend, John, sit down with me and tell me that I didn't look healthy. I was very unhealthy, and although I would wear a size 32 pants after this physical abuse, I looked horrible in them! As quickly as the weight fell, it came back even quicker, and each time there were more pounds added to the package. I overheard a coworker whisper, "Who pulled the rip cord on his ass?" This was accompanied with snickers and muffled laughs.

My tipping point occurred when I went to a medical clinic in Spain for a routine checkup. I instructed the nurse that we needed to take my blood pressure *before* my weight. She refused, saying, "That isn't how we do it here." She also refused to let me remove my shoes and perform the other customs and rituals that I had before a weigh-in. Then she had the height measure off center so I registered as very short (I am six feet or

183 cm). She had me as five nine! She entered all this numbers on my chart, tsk-tsked, and mumbled something about being obese. Then she took my blood pressure.

You can imagine—it was off the charts. I had walked into this clinic feeling I was a healthy normal guy and was leaving an obese midget about to explode from high blood pressure. I left the clinic with a prescription for blood-pressure medication and instructions that I would have to take these the rest of my life. The doctor smiled and said, "Oh, I know. It's so hard."

My blood pressure was averaging 160/106, and my cholesterol was close to 200. According to the norm, I was not considered to have high cholesterol yet, but I was dangerously close. Having a normal cholesterol reading, in a society where keeling over and dying of a heart attack is normal, is not such a good thing. Most heart attack patients fell within the normal or even optimal range.

After my appointment I began taking my blood-pressure medication. It did have some effects in the beginning. When I would reach for a book high on a shelf, I would get dizzy. I didn't feel as energetic as normal. There was one side effect that I was not expecting from this drug that I would have to take for the rest of my life. OK, so we all know that blood pressure lowers your "blood pressure." Men in particular have occasions where they would like a little pressure from Hemo the Magnificent. In other words, I was not able to "rise" to the occasion. Of course conventional doctors suggested that I counter this with prescription erectile dysfunction drugs. I was also told that at my age, sex was not as important. *What?* To whom? I did try the erectile dysfunction drugs and had a very rare side effect: blood in my ejaculate and preseminal fluid. Not a little, a great deal, and it was frightening. I wanted off the meds and to get healthy.

I began snoring loudly at night, huffing and puffing to get around, and breaking out into a sweat just from thinking! I remember my ninety-year-old father being worried that I would die before he did. I was fifty-six years old and functioned like I was eighty-six.

So this was the state of my body. I didn't feel that bad, and I was able to rationalize and excuse some of my situation to just be age related and normal. I had no idea that I could actually change everything and feel fantastic. I was, however, about to find out.

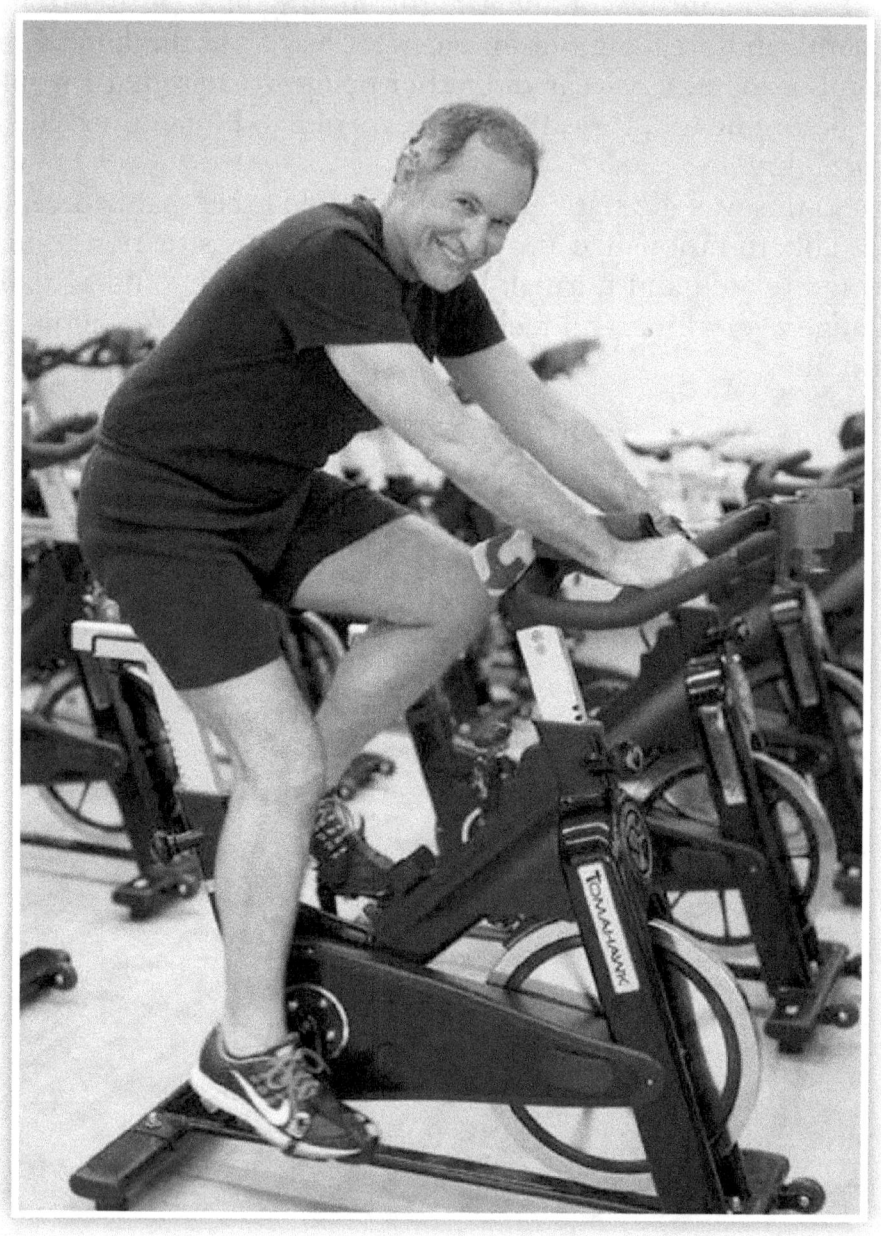

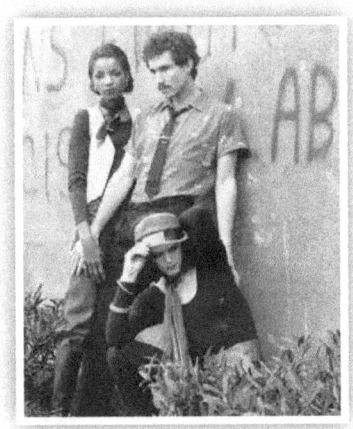

In this photo I managed to get to the weight required for the photo shoot: 145 pounds. I achieved this by swallowing wet cotton balls to reduce hunger. I was so unhealthy that my blood pressure dropped to dangerous levels, I had sores in my mouth and dark circles around my eyes, and my friends were warning me that I did not look well.

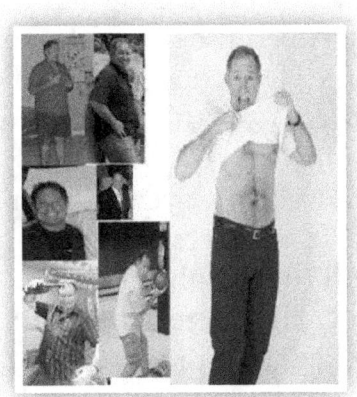

Before and after photos. My weight always bounced back after extreme dieting, but after starting a starch-centered diet, I lost seventy pounds, and it has not returned. My cholesterol dropped to 112, off all medications. Pants size from 38 to 32.

At all the support meetings from all groups, they tell you, "Inside every fat person is a thin person begging to be set free." I never believed that. Inside me was a fat slob growling, "Leave me the hell alone!"

So the answer was that I needed to get the weight off in order to get off the meds. Seemed simple. I just need to go on a diet. I decided to look at and review each diet I had tried in my life. Here is a list of diets that I can remember:

Three-Day Diet. Never seemed to get past day two. When I did get to day three, by day four, all the fat was back on.

Apple Cider Vinegar Diet. Felt like I burned a hole in my stomach. I wasn't hungry because I was sick to my stomach. The food plan was awful, and after I was done, I gained all the weight back.

Beverly Hills Diet. OK, this was insane. The watermelon day, I hurt from peeing all day. I ate everything and followed everything so I could get my free "golden pineapple" charm, which never arrived. It was a crazy pattern of eating, and after I was done, I gained all the weight back.

Blood Type Diet. Had to tell the clinic a crazy story to get my blood type checked; insurance companies were no longer paying for it, because it had become another fad diet. I ate everything that was perfect for my blood type. I didn't lose any weight. When I was done, I ate normally again and gained all the weight back. And then I gained some more!

Cabbage Soup Diet. The smell of that soup still haunts me. The concept is good, except you are hungry. The idea of eating a day of bananas or a day of meat is just a gimmick. The soup fills you up. If you follow the recipe exactly, it is really salty, and I did retain some water. When it was over my weight loss was modest. The mistake they make is to say, "Eat all the soup you want then eat a sensible meal." I ate tons of soup, and then I ate my meal. I lost only a few pounds, and I was miserable, gassy, and hungry. After I was done, I gained all the weight back, plus some.

Cambridge Diet. Drink-your-food concept. Lose the weight and then retrain yourself to eat sensibly. Here is the scoop. Your body shuts down into starvation mode, and then when you get off the liquid food and start eating real food, you gain lots of weight back. This is your body saying, "*Whoa*, you put me in a starvation mode again, I am sticking away some groceries for next time."

Dog Diet. The idea is eating only once a day, like a dog. Did you know Sumo wrestlers do this, too? I kinda ended up looking like one after this diet—well, in size, not in stamina or strength.

Atkins Diet. I did this diet a few times. Who could resist day one? By day three, my body was in ketosis,[1] and I felt horrible. My breath could stop a truck on the freeway, and my biggest pleasure in life was a poop, which happened rarely. I never lost a great deal of weight, but I did lose inches and patience with the general public. I gave up on the diet when I found myself crying and touching the potatoes in the grocery store. When I stopped the diet, I gained all the weight back and more.

1 Ketosis: The "ketogenic diets" cause the body to produce ketones by severe restriction of carbohydrate intake while allowing unlimited fat and protein intake. With insufficient intake of the body's primary fuel, carbohydrate, the body turns to fats from foods and from body fat for fuel. By-products of this metabolism are acidic substances called ketones (acetacetic acid, B-hydroxybuteric acid, and acetone). The metabolic condition is known as ketosis. Ketosis is associated with loss of appetite, nausea, fatigue, and hypotension (lower blood pressure). The result is a decrease in food (calorie) intake. Ketosis is the key to the diet's success, by allowing the body to starve while reducing the suffering of severe hunger pangs.

This same condition, ketosis, occurs naturally when people are literally starving to death or seriously ill. During starvation, this metabolic state is a kindness of nature, allowing the victim to suffer much reduced pains of hunger while dying. During illness the suppression of the appetite frees the person to rest and recuperate, rather than be forced by hunger to gather and prepare food. Because ketogenic diets simulate this metabolic state seen with serious illness, I refer to them as the "make-yourself-sick diets."

https://www.drmcdougall.com/health/education/health-science/featured-articles/articles/high-protein-diets/

Fit for Life Diet. To think that the only problem I ever had was that I was not combining foods right or eating them at the right time! I needed an app just so I knew when I could eat and what I could eat. "Want an apple?"

"Um, let me see. Oh drat, it's ten o'clock. I can't right now, but three forty-five would work. Or tomorrow." This is a life? I didn't lose anything, and I followed it to the letter…for, like, a day.

Fen-Phen Diet Pills. This is not funny. People died. I have a dear friend who also tried everything, and she started losing weight with fen-phen. Her husband loved her just the way she was, but she wanted desperately to lose weight. She died trying, literally. I had a physician who prescribed it for me. The first week I felt strange and could not sleep. I voluntarily stopped. I was one of the lucky ones. Not everyone was so lucky.

Fruitarian Diet. Ah, Woodstock and my repressed hippie loved this concept of eating only nature's fruit. "Just eat fruit, man, that's what God intended." Problem is that you are hungry. It is also not good for your triglycerides, and clearly we were not designed to just eat fruit. I did have a better understanding of why birds poop with any sudden movement.

Grapefruit Diet. Eat half a grapefruit before each sensible meal. "Sensible" should be changed to "small and boring." The idea is that the grapefruit has magical powers that change the food in our stomachs. I think the story of Jack's magical beans to find a golden harp is easier to swallow.

Jenny Craig. OK, she is just mean. I followed that plan to the letter. Met with my "personal" counselor once a week, whom I referred to as SB (Skinny Be-atch). She would approach the waiting room applying fresh lipstick, as I am sure she was purging her lunch before seeing me. She always would have me get on the scale, look extremely bored, and then sigh and say, "Well, at least we didn't gain, did we?" We? She wasn't there! OK, so you eat prepackaged food that tastes what I imagine army rations are like. I used to get the pancake mix, add it to the powdered eggs, mix them together to form a tortilla, add the chili in it to make an awesome burrito, and eat it with a salad. Sounds great, huh? It was edible. The only problem was that I had eaten my entire day's worth of food in one meal. Now I was back to the dog diet. You can't go anywhere. You just eat the prepackaged food with a few fresh vegetables. I was so excited for Wednesday. *Pizza!* I looked at that box, I caressed that box, I secretly kissed the box of pizza when no one was looking. I carefully placed her in the freezer to wait until Wednesday.

Wednesday arrived. I showered, put on nice clothes, and picked her up from the freezer. Greeted her with a big kiss and then heated up the oven. Oh yeah, baby. I carefully unwrapped the delicate package so I did not knock off one sliver of cheese or pepperoni. Once the pizza was completely "undressed," it was the size of an English muffin! I was starving after eating that minimorsel; I could have eaten the box. Yeah, I lost some weight, but I was hungry and felt deprived, and it felt like yet another failure in my life. After I was done, I gained all the weight back and then some.

Juice fasting with enemas and colonics. What says "vacation" like juice fasting and colonics? Kinda like summer camp for fat adults. I lost a great deal of weight during the seven days the first time and fourteen days the second time. I felt lighter than I had in years. It was the best feeling—for a week. Ohm, yoga, fasting, and a colonic twice a day to reduce the toxins in my body. The truth is, our bodies are releasing toxins all the time. We don't need to squirt water up our ass to get rid of toxins. Maybe it would be easier if we stopped putting the toxins in. As soon as I got home, I gained all the weight back and had a sore butt.

Last Chance Diet. Again, not funny. People died. You drink liquid, predigested protein for food until you reach your goal weight. I refuse to make a joke about the people who died. I was lucky. It is extremely hard on your kidneys and bones. After I was done, I gained all the weight back and quite a bit more.

Master Cleanse. Hey, Beyonce says it works for her, so it must be science. It is a starvation diet, and you lose more than fat. You lose muscle as well. Spicy-hot lemon water tastes awful, by the way. After I was done, I gained all the weight back.

Medifast. Liquid food diet. They now do this medically supervised, because anytime you do something this drastic to your body, there can be problems. Yes, I did it, because I was desperate for results. I hated having the body I had, and I also wanted to eat real food. I just felt that if I could get to my ideal weight, then everything would be OK. I would be sensible, and I would never get to the size I was again. That self-talk is a trap. I have been caught in that trap many times. Yes, I lost weight, but after I was done, I gained all the weight back.

Metrecal. This was like Slimfast, but in the early days. It is a meal replacement shake that you had three times a day. Then you had a sensible meal. Is it just me, or does the word "sensible" make you want to go eat a pizza? I am so sick of this overused diet-world word. After I was done, I gained all the weight back.

NutriSystem. Jenny Craig in a different box. I understand you don't have to attend meetings now and you can order your "rations" online. This is nice—you don't have to meet SB every week. Like the others, after I was done, I gained all the weight back.

Raw Food Diet. The idea was fascinating, sexy, and exciting. Eat all this wonderful raw food and get healthy. It is almost impossible to go out to eat on a raw-food diet and get anything other than a salad. Getting a "raw dressing" is impossible. Raw-food restaurants are very expensive because they are labor intensive. The food and recipes in general depend on eating a great deal of nuts, which are high fat. I rarely felt sated on this diet. I did lose some weight, and the weight gain was not drastic after I got off it. I ate lots of raw zucchini pasta with raw tomato sauce. I would get really full, but I was missing the feeling of being satisfied.

Scarsdale Diet. Oh look! The whole problem was that we were not combining foods correctly, and *that's* how we became such a fat nation. The claim that I could lose up to twenty pounds in two weeks was the hook. It has the "magical" combination of proteins and carbohydrates (Gasp! "Carbs" is a filthy word) that induces ketosis! In other words, another rework of the Atkins plan. So if I was seeking a near death experience, bad breath, and constipation, I could grab the meat and fat ring and go on a wild ride. Of course, the whole structure of the diet and the practicality of living it was impossible for me. I tried it and lost some and felt sick. After I was done with the diet, I gained the weight back in a matter of days—without trying.

Sego Diet Plan. This was a step up from the Metrecal diet I mentioned in the intro that I was on at age nine. And as a nine-year-old, I did lose weight pretty rapidly. For anyone who thinks my mom should not have given me this meal plan—She did it out of love. She did it because I would come home crying that the kids were picking on me. As soon as I lost some weight, I was taken out for a treat like a burger and fries and a milk shake! Once I stopped the structured eating, I gained all the weight back.

Slimfast. Same as Sego and Metrecal. Nothing new other than a different name and a celebrity thrown in to pitch it now and then.

South Beach Diet. Lists of acceptable and unacceptable foods, phase one, two, three, blah-blah-blah. Seemed like the only foods that tasted good were on the unacceptable list. The diet is seriously lacking in carbohydrates, which can put you in ketosis. I did not follow this diet for more than a day.

Sugar Busters. I liked the name of this diet. It had a Southern comfort feel to it. A friend from the South started me on this diet; she loved it. She followed it to the letter. She weighed almost four hundred pounds. Sometimes she would lose ten pounds! I tried it. Then I felt like I was being tortured on a sugar plantation and restricted from food. This diet is not too dissimilar to a diet that consists of following the glycemic index, though the Sugar Busters diet is more cut and dried. The theory is that spikes in your blood sugar are bad. *Hello*, our bodies are designed to eat food to raise our blood sugar, which turns off the hunger signal. Low blood sugar means we are hungry, and we eat to raise the blood sugar. With the Sugar Busters diet, all refined sugars are on the do-not-consume list. This includes anything with corn syrup, anything with molasses, all beer, all regular sodas, anything with dextrose, anything with glucose, and even regular honey. Given that a teaspoon of sugar only has sixteen calories, if it will get you to eat a nice healthful bowl of oatmeal, what is the problem? Then the plantation owner goes on to ban other carbohydrate-producing foods such as carrots, white rice, potatoes, corn, and anything with refined flour. Short-term weight loss, yes. Aftereffects weight gain? Yes.

Stillman Diet Plan. Another version of a ketosis diet. So again, you eat high-protein kidney-damaging meat, low-carbohydrate food plan that promises rapid weight loss in people who follow its rules precisely. I had to restrict my food intake to a narrow list of "approved" foods and beverages—mostly lean meats, eggs, and low-fat cheeses. I thought I really was going to outsmart this guy. See, he allows the use of a little mineral oil to prevent food from sticking to a pan. I decided to make mayonnaise the approved food and whipped up some fluffy mayonnaise using mineral oil. Tasted strange, but I was hungry. Have you ever heard of anal seepage? Nor had I. The mineral oil passes right through you and leaks out your butt. Mineral oil is not something you want to eat. Anyway, this diet sucked, just like the others.

Weight Watchers. This diet plan teaches us fatties how to have control and moderation. All in all, I have to say that the plan is OK, and their success rates speak well. I did get to meet others who struggle with weight loss and developed camaraderie without the consumption of food. I was not successful. The whole point system didn't work for me. I started playing the stock market with my points. In other words, I was buying futures. I attended my Wednesday meeting, and I was asked if I had a clue why I had gained a couple of pounds. Was I following the point system of twenty-five points per day? "Yes," I replied, "absolutely, but I kinda borrowed points from the other days, and technically I can't eat again until Sunday."

I have a dear friend who is a Weight Watchers counselor, and the program suits her well. I just am not the type who can be disciplined to only eat a certain number each day. So yes, I lost a little weight, but I can say that when I stopped this program, I didn't gain back as rapidly as after the others.

Zone Diet. Oh yeah, baby, I am in the zone! I love a gimmick that tries to distract me with time or fruit acid to avoid eating certain things. You see, according to this diet, food is like a drug and has to be taken at certain times. Right. You balance your food for the right proportions and can make sure your insulin and other inflammation-promoting hormones stay "in the zone," not too high or low, by eating foods at every meal in the right proportions: 40 percent carbs, 30 percent protein, and 30 percent fat. So one visit to a restaurant, and you are out of the zone. Then you start to just plain ZONE out on this whole thing, because it doesn't work for people who have lives or a human body. Have you ever taken a look at the doctors who write these books? Have they tried their diets? They don't look very slim, trim, or healthy.

I didn't even add the diets that I haven't tried, because they were just too far from science or nature. Paleo? What a joke! Why is it that they think prehistoric man ate meat all the time? Because they found arrowheads next to their bodies and no banana peels? Vegetables do decompose, ya know. Thanks to science, we have found that prehistoric people had fragments of starch in their teeth. Grain Brain and Wheat Belly are just revisits to the high-protein, low-carb diets that are not scientifically supported and are harmful.

I can tell you without a doubt and from my personal experience, diets in themselves—as a short-term fix—do not work. They actually *hurt* more than they help.

There are many reasons. I was still playing the recording that said, "Hey, you lost weight, now you can reward yourself." This example was clear at a Weight Watchers meeting when the leader asked, "How are we planning to handle

Thanksgiving, hmm? Christopher, how are *you* planning to manage Thanksgiving this year?" I looked at her and said, "With a fork and a knife. Why the hell you think I am here?" Clearly I had the wrong motivation. I was looking for a quick fix. I was the king of yo-yo.

At all the support meetings of all the groups, they tell you, "Inside every fat person is a thin person begging to be set free." I never believed that. Inside me was a fat lazy slob growling, "Leave me the hell *alone!*"

First, let's look at why. What happens to the pleasure center in our brain when we eat? Have you ever been on a diet and then one day scream, "Argh! I have to have a burger or chips," or something? Then society looks at you with a tsk-tsk and declares, "*You* didn't have willpower. *You* are a weak person."

I want you to know that isn't true. You are not! The pleasure centers in our brain are so strong that in laboratory experiments, rats would walk over live electrical wires in order to get the drug they needed to trigger their pleasure center, the same as drug addicts will give up food or caring for a child *just* to get their pleasure center triggered. This is not an excuse, but when you understand why your body seeks fat, it helps you understand your cravings.

Each time I tried a diet, I would tell my friends, "Oh, I can't go out with you this week. I'm on a diet, but next week I can." They would ask, "How long will you be on a diet?" No one ever treats a diet as a lifestyle change. We go on a diet, lose a few pounds, return to our old eating habits, and gain it back and even more. Our bodies are incredibly smart, and they will begin storing fat in case of another famine. We are creating mini-famines with traditional diets. Plus nothing really changes. We still view the diet as short term to "get control" of our bodies.

Cows are vegan, and you don't see any protein-deficient elephants! The overconsumption of proteins, especially animal-derived proteins, can have adverse health consequences.

My friends, family, and physician told me, "All things in moderation." My first response was, "Yeah, right, you are not exactly thin! None of you can take a flying leap through a clarinet yourselves." Oh, be careful—*very* careful—when insulting an F² (former fatty). We have had a lifetime of practice at hurling insults right back at ya!

I never really did anything with moderation, so who would think I'd to be able to eat food in moderation? When I smoked, I was not a social smoker who had two or three cigarettes in an evening. I had a pack and a half! I tried every brand, every shape, every flavor. I became a connoisseur. Yes, there are some people who are extremely disciplined and can do things in moderation. I cannot. I dive right in and do it to the max. There is a world full of humans who do the same.

CHEESE AND DAIRY

Cheese was my heroin. I had to have cheese. I thought I was self-righteous not eating dessert and just eating cheese for dessert. My favorite lunch? Homemade pimiento-cheese sandwich. Those of you who are not from Texas or the South, let me explain what this is. You get shredded cheddar cheese and add pimientos and mayonnaise and a little dash of Tabasco, and you are good to go. Only things missing are the cardiac paddles. Cheese, I felt, was vegetarian, and basically helping the environment and not harming animals. I loved cheese so much that I started making it at home. One time while making cheese, I decided not to salt the curds and see if I could make some kind of salt-free cheese. The results? Disgusting! So basically, you separate curds from the whey. Curds and whey—what could be more wholesome? We think of Little Miss Muffet and happy thoughts! The truth is, we are separating the fat from the milk. You have to add salt to the fat to make it taste decent. So really, do I love cheese, or do I crave and love the fat and salt? I think the answer was obvious by looking at my waistline.

Dairy is just liquid meat and not healthy for you. We are not designed to drink milk. For those of you who have been told that you need dairy for your bones, there are alternatives. Cow's milk was designed to grow a calf into a six hundred-pound cow. It works! I won't even get into the hormones, contaminants, pus (yes, pus), and other foul things in dairy.

First, excess protein from milk in your body is acidic and must be neutralized by taking calcium from your bones to neutralize the acid and flush it through your kidneys. So milk is not doing your body good. On top of these, people in the countries with the highest milk consumption have the highest incidents of hip fractures and osteoporosis.

BOOZE

OK, I listed this under moderation because, well, I used to drink lots and lots of red wine for my health, gin and tonic to party and be sociable, and Campari and soda for a sensible business-type meeting. In other words, I didn't drink with moderation either.

Three years ago, I could have written a book called *BoozyWhore*. Again, all of you perfect people say, "All things in moderation." Ha! I have held the hair of some of you "moderate drinkers" while you did the Technicolor yawn. I thought I did drink in moderation. In the doctor's office when they ask on the form, "How many drinks in a week?" I would look up at the ceiling, counting, tapping my pencil. When I had the real number, I thought, *Naah, that can't be right*, so I would put down a lesser number. I also knew never to get my liver function tested at the doctor's office without going three days without a drink.

I live in Europe, and Europeans drink all the time, right? No. The expats (expatriates) and visitors do. During the week, I would open a bottle of wine and share it with my partner. Half a bottle per person, right? That's two glasses per person. Seems that I ended up with three, and the other person with one.

In a group setting, it is easier. You look at everyone and say, "Red for the table?" When they all agree, then you can order away and not worry that anyone is really looking to see how many glasses you had, because when the bottle is empty, you just order more. I could tell how much wine I had by how I felt the next morning. I found that the more I drank, the less bad I felt the next day. It was kinda like training for a marathon or a drink-a-thon. I was never sloppy…well, rarely. Those of you who know me, shut up!

So after making the change to a starch-centered diet, did I give up drinking? No. Let me tell you how my drinking looks today. If I go out to a restaurant, I will order a glass of wine or a gin and tonic. I might have two. I try not to go out to a restaurant more than once a week, because it is difficult to find places that will not dump oil all over your food.

Recently, I did go to a favorite restaurant of mine in Nerja, Spain, called Lan Sang Thai. Amazing food, and they will make you a starchiwhore dinner! The staff knows me, and when I walked in, they asked if I wanted my "usual"—a Hendricks and tonic with cucumber. I had one, and then I had a second. The waiter reminded me that I normally had three. The next morning, I thought I was going to die. I was in pain and agony. My body was seventy pounds lighter, and my liver was not used to being flooded with this much poison to filter out. Lesson learned.

Bottom line is this: Alcohol will stop your weight loss. Alcohol lowers your inhibitions, which causes you to make bad choices. Alcohol is also a drug. A small amount to relax on occasion is OK. When alcohol becomes a focus, when you select restaurants or friends based on alcohol consumption or availability, then there is a problem. Alcohol causes other problems, like cirrhosis of the liver. This is the one item I have to toast to the self-righteous moderation people.

MEAT, CHICKEN, FISH, EGGS

My meals used to be centered on one or more of these. What's for dinner? Chicken! Oh, and did I remove the skin from roasted chicken? Absolutely, and slid that puppy right down my throat. I always felt I was doing well and being healthy by eating fish or chicken. I would remove the chicken skin and then cook it in a nice cheese and sherry sauce, just to be healthy. I remember my mom once critiquing me that I always prepared some type of sauce when I made steak. Either a red-wine reduction, green peppercorn, béarnaise, or something. She liked just a plain broiled steak with garlic salt. If you just boil meat in water, no one seems to like the flavor except for your dog or cat. Ever wonder why? Because our tongues and systems are not designed to seek amino acids like a dog or a cat. That is why we like BBQ sauce or other sauces on meat, poultry, or fish, because really, on their own they are not that flavorful.

Meat is also supposed to form our character. People will say, "I deserve a steak dinner." Real men eat steak! Real men die of heart attacks, too. Hey, meat builds muscle, and if you don't eat meat you will not be strong. If that were true, then everyone in the United States would be body builders. Why is it that athletes don't meat/protein-load? They carbo-load because they know what gives healthy energy. Eating meat does not translate into building muscle. We put salt on eggs or add mayonnaise and other items to make them tastier. We justify this because we have all been programmed that we *must* eat these items, or we will die from lack of protein. Do you know anyone with a protein deficiency? I know lots of people with problems with an overabundance of protein.

SO YOU'RE A VEGAN?

Most people say to me, "Oh, you're a vegan." The answer is no, but yeah, but no, but…yes, in a way. The problem I have with the term "vegan" is that it immediately focuses my diet on animal rights. Yes, that is a benefit to not eating flesh; however, the number one focus of my diet is my health. Also, there are many fat vegans. You can eat oil-laden processed food and declare yourself a vegan. Consume processed fake meats with isolated protein, and you are headed down the same unhealthful path you were on while eating flesh. Many vegan restaurants use isolated proteins to try to mimic meat products, and they add oil and more to try to make you think you are eating meat. The truth is that these processed, oil-laden foods may save a cow, but they will kill you in the process. Did you know that Oreo cookies, for example, are vegan? Potato chips, too. I could sit and eat bags of chips and cookies and then declare that I am overweight because of a vegan diet.

I am not a "raw" vegan because I do love cooked food. I do try to eat raw vegetables in some form every day, either as a salad or just as a snack. There are some raw vegan foods that are healthful, but most vegans rely on the addition of nuts and seeds, which are calorie-rich and very oily. I have made vegan raw-zucchini pasta with a spiralizer and a fresh tomato sauce that's wonderful! I also had a raw pesto made with avocado that was terrific, but I save avocados for special occasions or feast days. People who are looking to gain weight can eat more avocados than I can. Remember, the fat you eat is the fat you wear! Avocados are high fat and, like nuts, should be enjoyed in moderation on occasion.

So yes, I do not eat anything that poops or comes from an animal, so by that definition I am a vegan. I prefer being called a starchivore, because my focus is on health.

PORTION CONTROL

I do not like being PC in any form. Portion control, I was told, was the reason I was fat. The truth is that I was fat because I was hungry. Everyone wanted me to think it was because I didn't have any control. I was undisciplined. All the negative self-talk and others around me convinced me that must be the case. I would watch people eat small portions and then push their plate, eyes rolling, and exclaim, "Oh, I could not eat another bite! There is just entirely too much food." What was I thinking? I was thinking, *Pass that plate right over here, skinny be-atch, because I have my "eating pants" on.* I was hungry. I would eat more bread in a restaurant so I could feel full. Nouvelle cuisine? I thought that must be French for "small portions." Nothing worse than going out and spending a hundred dollars on a dinner only to return home and have a pimiento-cheese sandwich so I could sleep.

CALORIE IN, CALORIE OUT

Many people would tell me to just exercise more and eat less, that there is no magic bullet. I believed them. Notice I used the word "believed," because I know that isn't the case. The body is an amazing machine. It is built so that if we take in food, then our brain tells us when we have had enough. If a calorie is just a calorie, then a normal-size pimiento-cheese sandwich should tell my brain that I have had enough, and I should not be hungry. That isn't the case. Fat in our food goes immediately to fat cells and does not take up much room in your stomach. One small pimiento-cheese sandwich has 37 grams of fat and 560 calories. I could eat a huge bowl of mashed potatoes and fat-free gravy that would have 320 calories, 0.8 grams of fat, AND—are you ready for this?—8 grams of protein! My stomach fullness receptors would be triggered, and my brain would say, "OK, thanks, dude. We are ready to roll for a while now." So the type of calorie does affect how our satiety factor kicks in. Our bodies are designed to feel full then shut down our hunger. These diet advisers eat one cracker and smugly declare, "Oh, that is plenty for me, I couldn't *possibly* eat more." Meanwhile, these people drink their calories in a bottle of wine.

HERE I AM

So now you have an idea of how I got to where I was: overweight and unhealthy. I woke up every day ashamed and feeling guilty. I blamed genes, I blamed myself, I blamed my age, I blamed my life; I blamed anything I could because I just didn't understand how I could get like this. Why would God make me like this? I was not going to have my stomach cut, and I wanted to find something I could do and still enjoy my food. I decided to give Dr. McDougall and a starch-centered diet a try.

Potatoes with gravy, bean burgers with trimmings,
Corn soup and black beans, these are just the beginnings,
Bean burritos with salsa that is fit for kings,
These are few of my favorite things…
(sung to the tune of "These are a Few of My Favorite
Things")

HOW TO BE A STARCHIVORE

I am going to share with you how you can return to enjoying eating and no longer feel deprived or guilty about it. Imagine that! Whenever I ate in public, I always assumed people were looking at me in disgust, saying, "He really should not be eating that." Having guilt for partaking in one of the most important life-supporting activities is awful! It really is not your fault; it is the food. When you read about the magic bullet, I want you to be thinking of mashed potatoes and gravy, pasta with sauce, and comforting casseroles. It isn't about eating only vegetables.

Try this just for ten days and be amazed at the changes. Eat all you want of satisfying food and lower your cholesterol and your weight. After doing this program for ten days, I was off my blood-pressure medication. My cholesterol dropped, and I lost weight.

The dietary and lifestyle habits may sound challenging at first, but taken step by step over just ten days, it will become a way of life that is so natural that you won't believe how easy it is. Most important, you'll experience an almost immediate improvement in your health. And once you do, the profound difference will make it hard to imagine doing it any other way.

The diet, in detail, is available for free on www.drmcdougall. com.

Diet, however, is powerful medicine—if you're seriously ill or on medication, don't make a dramatic dietary change (or start an intensive exercise program) without the care of a physician who knows about nutrition and its effects on health. Never change medications without professional advice and, if appropriate, share this message with your doctor.

The Starch Solution uses a pure vegetarian diet based on starchy vegetables, plus fresh or frozen fruits and other vegetables. If you follow the diet strictly for more than three years, or if you are pregnant or nursing, take a minimum of 5 mcg (micrograms) of supplemental vitamin B12 each day.

THE FIRST TEN DAYS

The first ten days I was on this plan, it was really because I wanted to prove Dr. McDougall wrong, like all the other doctors. I wanted to show him that I could *not* eat all I wanted, lose weight, and gain better health. To make this a fair challenge, I did follow the diet to the strictest standards and did not deviate at all for the first ten days. I did not prepare anything with nuts, seeds, or avocados, which are higher-fat foods. I did eat lots of food. I was not hungry once. I ate bowls of brown rice with water-sautéed vegetables, vegetable broth, and a little hoisin sauce. I ate lots of mashed potatoes and gravy made with mushrooms and vegetable broth and thickened with brown-rice flour or sweet potatoes with a luxurious vegetable curry. I laughed as I ate to my heart's content, knowing full well that I was going to prove this doctor to be a yet another whack job. *Dr. McDougall is fit and trim*, I thought, *and he knows nothing about what it is like to be a struggling fat person.* I found out later this was not a true assessment.

The results after my ten days? First, my blood pressure went from 150/100 to 120/70. My cholesterol level dropped from 190 to 160, and I dropped four pounds. I felt fantastic physically, I had more energy, and I was pretty amazed, admittedly defeated that I could not prove Dr. Mc Dougall wrong.

Many people immediately discounted the diet having an effect on my blood pressure, stating that it was because of my weight loss. This is not true. My blood pressure dropped to normal in ten days. The only thing different that I did was stop eating the food that was causing damage.

I continued to follow this diet, and now, almost three years later, my weight loss is seventy pounds, my cholesterol is 112, and my blood pressure is 120/70. I feel fantastic. I am able to exercise as I never have before. My trainer actually has to tell me to rest and slow down!

I challenge you to try this diet for ten days. Try it in the strictest form for ten days. Meaning that "a little milk" in your coffee is not acceptable. Just give this a chance. Once you see and feel the difference, then make a decision.

You may find, as I did, that in the first few weeks, you are eating *tons* of food. I felt that there was something wrong because I was eating so much. There are a couple of things that are going on. One is that you will be developing flora to efficiently break down plant-based material, as opposed to meat and dairy. For me, flesh and dairy provided a different sensation of fullness in my stomach. You are also starving for clean natural food, and your body will respond with "Give me more!" Eventually, all of this changes, and you will naturally eat less because you are no longer hungry. I know some people who switched from a starch-centered diet back to eating meat, and they suffered stomach cramps and diarrhea. Your taste and cravings will change for clean, fresh, unprocessed food. Eventually, when you walk past the meat section of the store, you will actually wonder how people could consider eating that.

Remember that avocados, nuts, and seeds are high fat. Skip these for at least the first ten days. If you want to stop your progress with weight loss, eat a piece of avocado or a handful of nuts. This will halt your progress immediately! Although bread is allowed, limit your consumption because it is calorie dense.

During these first ten days, do not go hungry. Eat as much of the approved foods as you like. Have seconds if you want, and thirds. Do listen to your body and ask yourself if you are really still hungry. Clean out the junk food in your house and prepare food in case of cravings. What you will find is that starches are comforting. They are what our bodies crave.

BASICS

- A diet of plant foods, including whole grains and whole-grain products—such as whole wheat pasta, tortillas, and whole-grain bread, all without added oil or eggs—and a wide assortment of vegetables and fruit.
- Plenty of spices and usually small amounts of sugar and salt to enhance the flavor of food.
- Exercise—as simple as a daily walk.
- The exclusion of animal foods—red meat, poultry, dairy products, eggs, and fish—all of which provide toxic levels of fat, cholesterol, protein and, very often, infectious agents and harmful chemicals. So no red meat, poultry, dairy products, eggs, or fish.

- *The exclusion of all oils*, including olive oil, safflower oil, and corn oil. Oils are nothing more than liquid fats that increase obesity, which in turn depresses immune function and contributes to the most common chronic diseases. Even
- poly and monounsaturated fats—found in large amounts in vegetable oils and fish—have been shown to depress the immune system, increase bleeding, and promote cancers, especially those of the colon, prostate, and breast. Because all fats are easily stored by the body, too much dietary fat makes people overweight and lays the foundation for a host of other problems like heart disease, cancer, and adult-onset diabetes.

You will not be eating any dairy, meat, chicken, poultry, eggs, or meat by-products. You consume nothing that poops! Animal foods provide too much fat, especially the most harmful kind (saturated fat), which damages the arteries and causes heart disease and stroke. Beef derives 60–80 percent of its calories from fat; pork, 80–95 percent; chicken, 30–50 percent; and fish, 50–60 percent. Meat is also rich in cholesterol. A 3 1/2 ounce serving of beef contains 85 mg of cholesterol; pork contains 90 mg; mackerel fish contains 95 mg; turkey, 83 mg; tuna, 63 mg; and chicken (skinned, white), 85 mg. Our own bodies make all the cholesterol we need. You don't need to consume outside sources.

FOODS NOT ALLOWED
The following is a list of the foods that are not allowed on a Starch Solution Diet, with ideas for possible substitutions.

DO NOT EAT	POSSIBLE SUBSTITUTES:
Cow's Milk (for cereal or cooking)	Lowfat soy milk, rice milk, fruit juice, water, use extra when cooking hot cereal or pour over cold cereal
Cow's Milk (as beverage)	None; drink water, juice, herb tea, or cereal beverages
Butter	None
Cheese	None; after 10 days you may substitute soy- and nut-based cheeses
Cottage cheese	None; after 10 days you may substitute crumbled tofu
Yogurt	None
Sour cream	None for the first 10 days then you can substitute homemade tofu sour cream, not store brands (added oil).
Ice cream	Pure fruit sorbet, Frozen bananas, frozen juice bars; after 10 days you may substitute Lite Tofutti
Eggs (in cooking)	Ener-G Egg Replacer
Eggs (for eating)	None
Meat, poultry, fish	Starchy vegetables, whole grains, pastas, and beans; after 10 days you may substitute tofu "meat" recipes
Mayonnaise	Tofu mayonnaise
Vegetable oils (for pans)	None; use Teflon, Silverstone, or silicone-coated (Baker's Secret) or non-stick ceramic pots and pans
Vegetable oils (in recipes)	None; omit oil or replace with water, mashed banana, prunes or applesauce for moisture
White rice (refined)	Whole grain (brown) rice or other whole grains
White flour (refined)	Whole grain flours
Refined and sugar-coated cereals	Any acceptable hot or cold cereal. Oatmeal!

FRUITS AND VEGETABLES AS WELL!

Green and yellow vegetables are too low in calories to serve as the centerpieces of your meals but can be added without restriction. Start with a plain canvas like spaghetti and then add a rich vegetable marinara sauce or primavera sauce. Fruits—because they are high in simple sugars—should generally be limited to two servings a day, as they're tasty and easy to overconsume. The sugar in fruit is fructose which, for some, causes triglycerides and cholesterol to rise. People with these concerns should limit fruits even more. Dried fruit is concentrated fruit! It is easy to eat five hundred calories of fruit in a handful of dried fruit but much more difficult in fresh fruit. I personally limit myself to two fruit servings a day.

SO WHAT DOES A TYPICAL DAY LOOK LIKE FOR ME?

Breakfast is a bowl of oatmeal with a teaspoon of brown sugar sprinkled on top and a hot beverage.

Lunch is usually leftovers or homemade oil-free hummus with lettuce wrap or a sandwich made with oil-free hummus and roasted vegetables. For a quick and easy lunch, I put a scoop of cooked brown rice in a bowl, open a jar of beans and add in a quarter cup and a handful of fresh spinach, kale, or Swiss chard. Sometimes I make a sauce with a teaspoonful of mustard and a tablespoonful of balsamic vinegar. I have a rice cooker. You add the rice and water, and it stops cooking when it is done, and it holds the rice for thirty-six hours. You always have an emergency meal available. I freeze the leftover rice and use it for other things.

Dinner is usually seasonal vegetables in a sauce on couscous. Favorites include Moroccan vegetable tagine with preserved lemon and a few olives and raisins, and spaghetti and sauce with my "parmesan" sprinkled on top. I make it with a cup of almond meal, a cup of nutritional yeast, and a packet of instant miso soup powder. This mixture will last me about a month.

Dessert: Not a big one in our house, but on occasion we will have a fruit cobbler or frozen-banana ice cream.

Snacks: Air-popped corn, corn cakes, or soup.

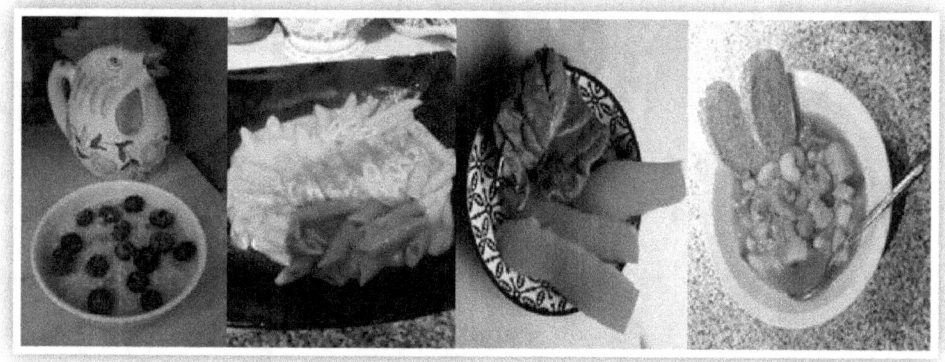

Here is a typical day: oatmeal with blueberries, whole-wheat macaroni and "pleeze," salad and a Spanish potaje (bean-and-vegetable soup) with multigrain bread.

Multiuse cooking: To save time, for a base I will prepare a large pot of something such as a large pot of plain lentil beans. The first day I will make a batch of lentil burgers for dinner and freeze a few for another time. The following day, I may make a hearty lentil soup, and the last day, puree lentils with some "hunky beefy stock" to make a base for a stew. I toss a bag of frozen stew vegetables or just chop up some, steam them, and stir them into the stew base. Voilà! A batch of kidney beans can be bean burgers, Italian pasta salad with kidney beans, and for day three, a kidney bean loaf with brown gravy. With a batch of pinto beans, I can have Mexiburgers, bean enchiladas and mashed beans and rice.

Pressure Cooking: I have always been terrified of pressure cooking. Today you can purchase electronic pressure cookers that are safe and foolproof. I place my beans in the pot and cover with water, and the following day I can cook a pot of beans in seventeen to twenty minutes. No time to presoak? You can pressure cook beans raw with water in thirty-five minutes.

Rice Cooker: This is the best invention! You add equal parts rice and water (I add a little more water with brown rice) and press on. The cooker stops when the rice is perfect, and the rice is held at a perfect temperature for thirty-six hours!

If you are struggling with an idea of what to prepare for the first ten days, here is a link for a sample of a ten-day meal plan: https://www.drmcdougall.com/health/education/free-mcdougall-program/10-day-meal-plan/.

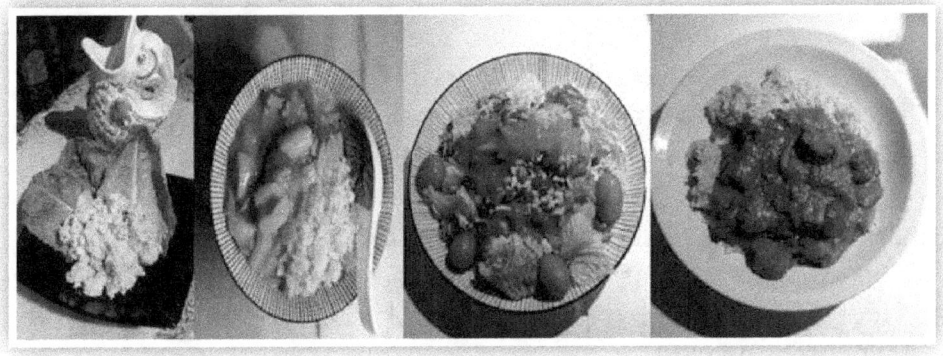

A few more examples are potato salad made with a homemade tofu mayonnaise, chickenless a la king with brown rice, vintner's salad with an oil-free pear vinaigrette, and mushrooms bourguignon and brown rice. All of these meals are superfast and easy. Find what you like and repeat it. Often we have beans and rice in tortillas and salsa.

COFFEE

I am originally from Seattle, and I love my coffee. I speak Starbucks and can order with the pros. Coffee is one of the things that I try to eliminate in my diet because of my history with high blood pressure. There are other reasons as well, but I won't get into them now. I have tried eliminating coffee from my diet in the past. As I mentioned, I don't do anything in moderation. I was drinking espresso twice a day during the week, and on weekends I used my special machine that would grind the beans and brew a perfect java. I tried slowly reducing my intake by changing the beans—two-thirds coffee and one-third decaf, then half and half. Finally, one-third real and two-thirds decaf, and *ding, ding, ding*! I was on full decaf without any withdrawal.

I went to my local coffee hangout, and they made a mistake and gave me full-on French roast full-caffeine coffee. I felt like a million bucks! However, I was right back where I started. As for me, I just don't go into a coffee place, or I order sparkling water. As for those moderation people, I am sure you have your coffee intake down to a science. That is great for you. Hip, hip, hooray for your self-control.

During the first ten days, if you can try to reduce or eliminate coffee, it is best. I don't want you to get withdrawal headaches and interpret it to mean that it is the diet causing you not to feel well. There are many herbal coffee substitutes available. Herbal teas as well.

Hotdog connoisseurs can eat pig anus, but offer them a vegetable version, and they shriek, "EEW!"

M any big companies are seeing the shift away from meat consumption, and they are making tons of fake meats. *Eureka!* I thought. *This will be easy to do. I'll just substitute all the bad things that I used to eat with these good fake things—fake hot dogs, hamburgers, ground beef, chicken, and more.*

Here is the problem with these products. They are highly processed soy and other protein isolates. They are manipulated and chemically changed to look and taste like meat products. They add fats, oils, and refined sugars to make them palatable. The frightening part is that these Frankenstein food products are more harmful than eating the real thing. I know one person who thought she was following the plan by eating Frankenweenies, and her cholesterol levels increased, and she gained weight. These aren't foods. Don't eat them.

The least of the bad is seitan, which is derived from the protein portion of wheat. You get dough and wash it until all that is left is the wheat protein. In the Seven Day Adventist church, I have seen recipes for this called "Do-Pep." This is still processed but to a lesser degree. If you want the protein from flour, then eat a piece of bread.

Yes, I love burgers, and I make them all the time. A combination of coarsely mashed beans, water-sautéed onions, and some spices, mixed with raw oatmeal and allowed to sit, will make excellent burgers. Hot dogs can be made by marinating whole carrots and cooking them in the marinade. And voilà you have a dog ready for the trimmings! There are several burger recipes available. Just be sure not to add any oil.

I do have a cheese recipe that I use only on special occasions that I will share. This is a variation of Mary McDougall's cheese sauce.

Melty Cheese Sauce
1/4 cup raw cashews
1 cup steamed cauliflower or roasted butternut squash (In an emergency, you can eliminate this ingredient, but it won't be as yummy.)
3/4 cup water
4 ounces pimientos
1/4 cup nutritional yeast
3 tablespoons cornstarch
1/2 teaspoon salt

Place all the ingredients in a blender and process until completely smooth. If you own a Vitamix, this process will take 3 minutes; if you own a regular blender, the process will take about 5 to 6 minutes.

Pour the mixture into a saucepan and cook at medium heat until the sauce thickens, about 5 minutes. Stir constantly.

This cheese sauce is great on just about anything. Pour it over a baked potato, have it on top of your favorite chili or over some baked tortilla chips. You can add in some chopped jalapeños or habaneros (if you like it hot and spicy), cumin, and a dash of chili powder to make a wonderful Mexican dip.

VEGETABLE BROTH

You will be using lots of vegetable broth. Be sure to read the labels on the brands you buy. You will be amazed how many use some milk product or added oil. I make my own concentrated vegetable bouillon in frozen cubes. I just pop a few from the freezer into the dish or in water, and I am ready to roll. This vegetable broth is so amazingly easy!

No Feathers Chickenlike Stock

2 medium carrots cut into chunks
1 large onion cut into quarters
2 stalks celery chopped coarsely
1 teaspoon poultry spice or 1/2 teaspoon sage or 1/2 teaspoon rosemary
3 springs fresh parsley or 1 1/2 teaspoons dried
2 sprigs fresh thyme or 1 teaspoon dried
1/2 teaspoon black pepper
1/2 teaspoon salt
1/2 cup water
1/2 cup nutritional yeast

Place everything except the nutritional yeast into a Crock-Pot or slow cooker. Cook on low for 8–10 hours. I usually place everything in here before I go to bed and then turn it on, and it is ready in the morning. No need to worry if it goes for 12 hours. It is not going to be overdone!

In the morning or after this has cooked, remove the thyme sprigs (if you used fresh). Now add the contents of this into a blender or food processor. I use an immersion blender, which works, but the results are not as smooth. Add the nutritional yeast and blend until as smooth as possible.

I pour into a container what I think I will use for the week, and the rest I pour into silicon ice-cube trays and freeze. If a recipe calls for one bouillon cube, I use two of mine, because it is not as concentrated as the commercial kind, and it contains no MSG or other chemicals. This is easy to make and tastes great. Good to have on hand.

Hunky Beefy Stock
1/2 cup dried mushrooms
1 large onion, cut into quarters
4 cloves garlic
1 cup water
1 teaspoon vegan Worcestershire sauce
1 teaspoon soy sauce

Process dried mushrooms in a spice grinder or food processor until it is a powder.

Place everything in the slow cooker. Cook on low for 8–10 hours. I usually place everything in here before I go to bed and turn it on, and it is ready in the morning. You don't have to worry about it getting overdone!

In the morning, or after this has cooked, put the contents into a blender or food processor. I use an immersion blender, which works, but the results are not as smooth. If a recipe calls for one bouillon cube, I use two of mine.

Starchiwore Mushroom Gravy
2 cups cold water or cold vegetable broth
1/4 cup white wine
1 Onion chopped
1/2 Pound sliced mushrooms
2 Tablespoons Corn Starch or Brown Rice Flour*
3 Tablespoons Soy Sauce

Spices: Add your favorites! I use parsley and thyme and black pepper. You could add basil or oregano or any combination you like.

Put wine and chopped onion in a sauté pan and sautee in the wine until the onions are soft. Add Mushrooms. Stir cornstarch into water or broth until dissolved. Pour stock and soy sauce into the pan and stir until the mixture is heated thoroughly and thickened.

*I love to use brown rice flour because you can add it to hot sauces and it will not lump. If you can't find brown rice flour at the market, you can make it in your blender! Add brown rice and blend on the highest setting until it is flour.

STARCH SOLUTION DIET MEAL PLANS

https://www.drmcdougall.com/health/education/free-mcdougall-program/10-day-meal-plan/

MY FAVORITE RECIPE LINKS

On www.drmcdougall.com are tons of recipes—over four thousand. Find a few that look good and prepare them! I am giving you a few of my favorite recipe links as well.

www.ImaStarchivore.com

https://www.drmcdougall.com/health/education/recipes/

http://blog.fatfreevegan.com/

http://engine2diet.com/recipes/favorites/

http://happyherbivore.com/recipes/

The most I learned from the lesson was this simple fact: if cheese and dairy weren't good for my cholesterol or blood pressure, and I didn't want to take medication or put myself at risk for a heart attack or stroke, I needed to stop eating cheese and dairy.

Sometimes we eat to celebrate. We eat out of boredom, or we eat out of depression. We eat for emotional reasons, not just physical. I use the word "we," and I really mean "I." Maybe you don't eat for these reasons. I know I do. Our culture focuses main events around food. It is difficult not to see food in ways that are not really necessary.

Depression was a big one for me. I used to eat when I was happy, but I gorged when I was depressed or frustrated. I could eat enormous amounts of food. I tried going to salad bars to binge, but I was never really satisfied until I started eating the pizzas offered at the buffet. Why? The carbohydrates in the bread was satisfying me, not the volumes of food. Eating a starch-centered diet allowed me to eat until satisfied. I did not feel guilty because I was still on the plan, and the carbohydrates increased serotonin levels, which affect mood and reduce appetite. It is a symbiotic relationship that works.

The biggest challenge on a starch-centered diet is not the food, but rather the people around you. The fact that you are eating in a manner that is different from the norm can actually make some people quite angry, especially because you are eating *carbs*. They act like it is a zombie apocalypse. Watch out!

There are the carb-eating zombies! It can also make them re-evaluate how they are eating or their health, and they may get angry with you.

The most common challenge you will hear is, "Where are you getting your protein?" When you tell them you get it from plants, it just doesn't connect. For fun, I look them in the eye and say, "Human flesh." I try to decide if they truly want to know and are interested, or if they are just challenging your newfound health and success. If they seem to really want to know, I will discuss where we get protein from and compare us to other species, like chimpanzees or apes, who are herbivores. I will share that the protein content in a potato or a bowl of rice is sufficient.

I also will ask them what the perfect food for human growth is. This usually prompts a blank stare, and to allow them to save face, I will answer, "Mother's milk, of course," with which they agree. I ask them the percentage of protein in mother's milk, which they don't know. I tell them that it is 5 percent protein. Next, I ask what the protein percentage is in a potato. They can't answer, and I assist with, "It is 5 percent as well." This usually will cause some discomfort, because it is breaking from the normal pattern.

Often your foes will say, "That is too much starch! You will get your blood sugar too high." Interesting argument, because that is the purpose of food. When we have low blood sugar, we eat to raise the blood sugar for energy. Complex carbohydrates like potatoes slowly release the sugars to provide energy, as opposed to table sugar, which raises the sugar rapidly. But then it drops to low levels again.

When you start this plan, and your friends find out, the first fear that crops up is failure. I used to think, *My friends are going to view this like a yogurt maker. Give it two weeks, and it's history.* I also had the fear that my friends would no longer invite me to their house or invite me to join them to restaurants. I had to plan in advance how I would tackle these challenges so when faced with them, it was a breeze. So many friends would present something to me and say, "I want you to just have a taste of this, for me. A little won't hurt." I would reply, "You know, that looks absolutely fantastic, and I am sure it tastes wonderful. However, as you know, I had to change what I eat for my health. If I could eat just a piece, I would not have gotten to the point where I did. Think of it as offering an alcoholic a drink."

I also make an effort to always make positive comments about what other people are eating. Some feel guilty that you are eating healthfully, but they have a steak and baked potato with sour cream on their plate. They *know* that what I am eating is better for them. They can see the results. I don't need to make them uncomfortable. I am always open to answer any question someone might ask if I think they genuinely want to know about a starch-centered diet.

The biggest challenge you are going to face is with yourself. Remember all that self-talk we learned growing up fat? Those thoughts will sabotage us. You know, like

- my family is all large. It's in my genes;
- I really am not that large. I am normal in size for my age;
- my partner said s/he would not be attracted to me if I were thinner;
- I don't want people to think that I am ill if I lose too much weight;
- I am perfectly healthy now. I don't need to make a change;
- if this was right for me, my physician would have suggested it long ago;
- my glands prevent me from losing weight, so why bother?
- I am just curvy—or stocky—regardless of what the charts show;

- I don't have time to prepare food. I am too busy making a living;
- the holidays or other events are coming around, and I will get back on track once that is over;
- I am a social person, and this just gets in the way and creates problems;
- I just read that there is a scientific report that says drinking wine every day and eating oil is good for me;
- I could never learn to like this food;
- it is not manly or ladylike to eat this way;
- my family would never do this, and I am not going to prepare two dinners or create problems for them. It upsets my family too much that I am eating this way, and they worry; and
- this just will get in the way of my social life.

If they are your friends, they want you to be healthy. If you are invited over for dinner, explain that your doctor has you on a special diet and offer to bring a dish to share. I have attended dinner parties where I brought my own entrée, and the host provided a simple salad. Many people were curious and wanted to taste what I was having. It is a great way to introduce your new way of living to others.

I will go ahead and go off this regimen for a few days and then return to it; I know I can. (I have encountered many starch-centered success stories who got cocky with the results and thought they had it managed, and they gained the weight back when they returned to unhealthy food.

Suppose something occurs, and you want to binge. Rather than use your favorite binge food, find another. Mine? Mashed potatoes with mushroom gravy, or beans and rice on a corn tortilla with melty cheese sauce (I share the melty cheese sauce recipe in the book).

The main key to these thoughts is the fear of change. If you can commit to a month of eating a starch-centered diet, after you experience the changes, you won't want to go back to unhealthful eating. After two years, you will wonder how anyone can eat the unhealthful way. You are going to feel incredible and appreciate how much better that feels than sick. I didn't really think of myself as sick until after eating a starch-based diet, and then I was shocked by how much better I felt. Each day you will lose a little more weight, you will feel better, you will be more energetic and confident.

Bad days happen. For all of us. When they occur, what I think about is: How am I feeling right now on a scale of one to ten, ten being fantastic? If I am at a five, I ask myself, "If I had a magic wand and made a change, right now, what would that change look like? (OK, of course I say I want to be a fit body builder *right now*, but that isn't going to happen. Make it realistic.) Ask yourself, "What can I do to make it a six right now"? I continue through this process until I can find a manageable and tangible way to make a change that does not sabotage my success.

Another big challenge is what to do if you are in a situation where you can't follow the plan. This should be a *rare* occurrence if you plan in advance, but sometimes it can happen. Here is what I suggest. Have a predetermination plan, meaning a contract that you make with yourself for what to do if you have a slipup.

My Predetermination Plan

In the event that I find myself in a situation where I cannot stay with the plan

1. I will not beat myself up and give up;
2. I will immediately return to the plan;
3. I will not allow myself more than one cheat meal in a week;

4. I will not use this as an excuse not to follow the plan;
5. I understand that the forbidden food may make me not feel well;
6. I will remember how good I felt when I was on the program; and
7. _____ (customize to what works for you).

This contract with yourself is to help keep you on track. It is too easy to say, "Forget it," and fall face first into a cheese pizza!

DISPELLING COMMON MISCONCEPTIONS

Some people are hesitant to fully embrace a starch-centered diet because the information is different from what they have heard, and thus they are afraid. They're afraid they won't get the nutrition and protein, or that it might be too expensive, or they just won't have time to prepare everything.

A whole-food, plant-based diet is too expensive—At first glance, fast-food hamburgers are a lot cheaper than a salad, but let's look at some facts. While specialty plant-based convenience foods can be sometimes pricy, if you select whole-food choices, you will get much higher nutritional value for your money. For example, beans, other legumes, and whole grains are a lot less expensive than meats, and they're loaded with protein, vitamins, and minerals. And if you buy them in bulk, they will be less expensive.

Buying fruits and vegetables that are in season from your local farmer's market is a much better value than the supermarket most of the time, and the produce is often fresher and usually naturally ripened (instead of being picked prematurely and ripened in the back of a semitruck on the way to the store.) Do you even remember the smell of a vine-ripened tomato?

When you buy flash-frozen off-season fruits and vegetables, you will often get many more nutrients than from fresh vegetables and fruits that are picked prematurely. Frozen fruits and vegetables have the added benefits of being not only convenient but much more economical.

My grocery bill is a fraction of what it used to be. We calculated that we save almost $2,000 a year since switching to a starch-based diet.

Incomplete protein with a starch-based diet—A common question is, "Where do you get your protein?" I get so tired of hearing this. The old reply is standard. "Plants don't supply 'complete' proteins" All plants contain all of the amino acids in proper balance for ideal human growth. It is impossible to make up a diet deficient in protein or individual amino acids from any unrefined starches (rice, potatoes) and vegetables. The only real problems with protein come from eating too much, usually the result of a diet high in animal foods.

Proteins are made from chains of twenty different amino acids that connect together in varying sequences. Plants can synthesize all of the individual amino acids that are used to build proteins, but animals cannot. There are eight amino acids that people cannot make, and thus, these must be obtained from our diets—they are referred to as "essential."

Since plants are made up of structurally sound cells with enzymes and hormones, they are by nature abundant sources of proteins. In fact, so abundant are plants that they meet the protein needs of the earth's largest animals: cows, elephants, and hippopotamuses, for example. You would be correct to deduce that the protein needs of relatively small humans can easily be met by plants. As long as you're taking in enough calories from whole foods, you're taking in plenty of protein.

You are eating too many carbs and you are going to get fat—Carbs are not the zombie food they've been made out to be. Fruits, vegetables, and whole grains are high in complex carbohydrates, which is what your body needs for energy. Whole, plant-based foods are rich in necessary vitamins, protein, minerals, and antioxidants; they are high in fiber as well. Fiber helps slow the digestion of carbohydrates. This means you don't experience the bad effects of processed (or stripped) carbs, like a candy bar or a sugary soda, that make your blood sugar spike and then plummet. Look at countries whose population eats a starch-centered diet. They are slim. You may argue that it is genetics. If this were the case, then explain why when they change to a Western-type diet, they all get fat and develop illnesses associated with a Western diet? It's the food!

Eating a starch-centered diet takes too much time—This just isn't the case. In the time it takes for you drive to a fast-food restaurant and bring home a steaming-hot artery-clogging dinner for your family, you could have prepared a healthful starch-centered meal. Preparing healthful whole-food meals doesn't mean you'll be chained to the stove for eternity. Keep it simple when you're pressed for time. You can steam vegetables like squash or broccoli in less than ten minutes, including prep time. Invest in a rice cooker. There's nothing like a perfect rice without the worry. Put the rice in, add water, and press on. It stops when the rice, couscous, quinoa, or other grains are ready and holds them at serving temperature for thirty-six hours. Use your slow cooker. You can cook everything from soup to beans to enchiladas and quinoa in a slow cooker. Toss everything in the pot before you leave for the day, and dinner will be waiting for you when you get home. Another great way to integrate a whole-food, plant-based diet is simply to plan ahead with a weekly menu and stock your pantry or freezer full of dinners. I always prepare more than needed and freeze the leftovers.

You are going to be hungry all the time—That is just not the case at all. A whole-food starch-centered diet can be totally satisfying. If you are eating plenty of whole-food plant-based foods, you will be loading up on fiber. Fiber is really what makes you feel satiated; it fills up your stomach and stabilizes your blood-sugar levels to prevent cravings. Legumes (beans, peas, and lentils) are particularly good because they are composed of hunger-satisfying protein and have uniquely high levels.

With a starch-based diet, you might have to shop a little differently, think a little more about the variety of foods you include in your diet, and spend a few more minutes in the kitchen, but in the end, you will reap enormous slimming and nutritional rewards.

Give it a try. You'll soon discover that you feel so fantastic, you're healthy, and your friends are commenting how well you look that you could not imagine going back to your old way of unhealthful eating.

THINK THROUGH YOUR DAY

I think about what I am going to do for the day, and I plan out my food. For example, if I am going to be out running errands and will not be able to be home for lunch, I will grab a couple of potatoes, put them in one of those Potato Express bags for the microwave (brilliant product), cook them for eight minutes, pop them in a bag, and bring them with me. If I get hungry, I can take out a potato and eat away! The bags steam them, and if you have a Yukon Gold potato its taste is almost buttery. In my village in Spain during sweet potato season, a vendor will sell me a freshly baked candy-sweet potato that I can eat as I walk.

Where you get into trouble is being hungry without options. I try to always have a backup plan. If I know I am going to a restaurant with friends, and there will be only a few options for me, I have something in the refrigerator ready for when I return home. Sometimes I eat before I go out. So the most important thing to do is plan your day and follow your plan.

PORTIONS

Eat as much as you want. Just don't be hungry. The first few days, you may find yourself eating more than normal of a variety of delicious food. Part of it is that your body is excited to be flooded with nutrients and healthful food. Another aspect is that the sensation of fullness is different than when you eat a meat- and dairy-heavy diet. I have witnessed people eat huge amounts and still lose weight. Granted, these people had more weight to lose than others. A technique that my trainer, Fran, used to teach me about my PC (portion control), was to take a photo of each and every meal and item I ate in a day. I had to send these to him. By the end of one week, I could see that I was eating larger portions than were necessary for my age and activity level. This visual was a huge help in getting me to eat normal portions yet not be hungry.

PLATEAU

How much weight you need to lose will determine the rate of weight loss. I lost weight quickly the first few weeks, and then it slowed down to maybe a pound a week. As I approached my ideal weight, I stopped losing. I had a final ten pounds to go. As you approach your ideal weight, the process is much slower, but there are a few things you can do to get those last few pounds off. One is to eat smaller portions but extend it through the day. The idea is that you feed your body enough for energy so your body will release stored fat, knowing that more food is on the way. There is an extreme example of this at the end of this book. The other, my preferred choice, is to go on a "Mary Mini" which is listed at the end of this book.

GAS

Some of you may ask if this way of eating will cause gas. Bowel gas is produced by the action of intestinal bacteria on foods.

Carbohydrates that have not been absorbed in the process of normal digestion by enzymes in the small intestine are moved undigested into the large intestine (colon), where bacteria break them down by fermentation, which creates gas! You all who have attempted to make beer or wine at home know this one well. The gas that is produced is actually five gases: nitrogen, oxygen, hydrogen, carbon dioxide, and small amounts of methane. These account for 99 percent of bowel gas. These gases are odorless. The strong odor of bowel gas comes primarily from products of bacterial putrefaction of animal proteins and fats in the large intestine, so avoiding animal products in your diet means cleaner and fresher air.

The number-one source of undigested carbohydrate is lactose from dairy products, such as milk, skim milk, and yogurt. The second leading gas-producing foods are legumes, whether they come as beans with hot dogs, or in a low-fat vegetarian chili. They contain two relatively indigestible sugars that end up in the large intestine, where they are decomposed into gases by bowel bacteria.

You are also now going to be eating a high-fiber diet. Your body needs time to adjust and grow new bacteria to minimize gas. Within two weeks your gas will be diminished to normal. The biggest difference is that when you do pass gas, it will not be the odoriferous, clearing-out-the-room kind of gas. Just a nice little puff of starchiness. If you know a particular food causes you gas, then avoid these foods and incorporate them slowly to see how you adjust.

Everyone seems to have some kind of method to remove gas from beans. I have tried them all. I have personally found that precooked canned beans often will give me gas. My home-cooked beans do not. My theory is that in mass production in the canning process, not all the sugars in the beans are cooked out; therefore, they ferment in the gut, causing gas. Some claim that sprouting beans before cooking will reduce the gas as well. Cover the beans in water for twelve hours. Then spread the soaked beans on a wet towel until you see small white shoots appearing. This means they are using their sugars for sprouting. Cook the beans, and you may find less gas.

TRACKING YOUR PROGRESS

In the beginning, it is handy to keep detailed records—of meals, exercise regimen, physical status (including symptoms that have disappeared), mental status, test results, and medications—in order to track your progress. Take as many body measurements as you can on the first day of the program, and then take those same measurements again on the last day. An activity tracker is helpful to keep you moving. Set a goal and take a look to see where you are. Get up and go for a walk or go out in the garden. Even housework will trigger activity.

Whenever possible, track at least the following basics: your weight, your blood pressure, and blood test results, including the five measures below, plus any additional recommendations from your doctor. I personally recommend that when you start this diet you have your B12 checked. Then you will have a baseline to show your B12 levels before the diet, in case your physician has a notion that your B12 is low after doing this plan.

- **Cholesterol**: If your level is above 180 mg/dl, you should consider it a warning sign of potential circulatory problems. Ideal is below 150 mg/dl. Sometimes results are broken down into HDL ("good") and LDL ("bad") cholesterol levels, but I feel total cholesterol is the most significant.
- **Triglycerides**: This measures the amount of fats floating in your blood. Your level will likely be between 50 and 200 mg/dl. Higher levels indicate "sludge" in your

blood, cause resistance to insulin activity, and are associated with an increased risk of heart disease.

- **Glucose (blood sugar) level**: Normal *fasting* level is between 70 and 100 mg/dl. Higher levels indicate prediabetes or diabetes.
- **BUN (blood urea nitrogen)**: This level reflects the amount of protein you eat and the function of your kidneys. Normal is less than 15 mg/dl.
- **Uric acid level**: Normal is less than 7 mg/dl. A higher figure indicates a risk of developing gout and/or kidney stones.

Having a "normal" cholesterol in a society where it is normal to keel over of a heart attack is not a good thing! Most heart attack patients fell within the normal cholesterol range—even the optimal range.

I am adding this part because many physicians do not understand nutrition. They often are operating from the same information that we are. I recall seeing one medical booklet on nutrition in my father's office. I thought it was amusing that it was written by an organization that promotes meat and dairy consumption. Most physicians receive little education on nutrition. They are well versed in other areas, but nutrition is not one that is a focus in medical school. Pharmacology, yes, nutrition, no. Many of you will be sharing your desire to change your diet with your physician. For this reason I added this chapter. I have seen people achieve great results on a starch-centered diet only to be told by their physician that they are better off just taking pills to combat the effects of eating artery-clogging foods.

Where to start. First, my father was a doctor in a small town in Texas, and he was well respected. Doctors do study a great deal, and they should be applauded for their hard work. There are several highly qualified, respectable physicians in the world. There are also some who could use additional continued education and customer service training.

You need a physician who understands your desires. For example, my physician knows that I prefer to be healthy, not take medications. My physician knows that I eat a starch-centered diet. My physician also knows that he needs to explain to me *why* he is making a recommendation and what medical evidence he has to support that decision. I have fired a physician for saying that I couldn't understand, or "Because I am a doctor," to which I replied, "I am the paying customer."

Once I had the opportunity to sit in with a patient who was ninety years old. The physician was gushing over her blood results and general health. He then turned to me and asked, "What do you think?" I replied that yes, she was looking fantastic for ninety; however, I didn't feel a blood cholesterol of 200 mg/dl was anything to celebrate when we know that there are no cardiac occurrences in patients with a total cholesterol under 150. Also, the patient reported that she was taking a powerful laxative three times a week, and from reviewing what she was consuming, it appeared that a higher-fiber starch-centered diet would 1) reduce the total cholesterol, 2) reduce or eliminate her need for laxatives, and 3) reduce her arthritis pain.

I added, "Furthermore, doctor, I appreciate your suggestion that she eat dried fruit, but she reports that she drinks two Diet Cokes a day and not much more liquid. Don't you think we are exacerbating her condition? Maybe eating the whole fruit would have more of a benefit. She needs water."

The physician responded in a condescending manner, "Are you a physician? What qualifications do *you* have?"

I replied, "I have a library card, and the information is available to anyone." This prompted his reply that there is absolutely no clinical evidence that changing diet in a patient this age would help anything. I referred to a study by the Arthritis Association and he dismissed it, saying that was from the eighties (as if the information has changed?). I did not want to make the situation any more uncomfortable than it was, and I left it.

I don't want to appear combative and preachy. I am trying to encourage people to take control of and accountability for their own health. While consulting a physician is a good idea, it is not the be-all and end-all to being healthy. In fact, shopping for a doctor is as important as shopping for a mate. Even you have a doctor who works with your health goals, it is still OK to challenge them. While they have attended school for years and do require ongoing education, they are not omniscient, and there is no way they can know everything and how it will affect your body.

Often we are left to our own defenses. No one is more interested in you than you are. Therefore, you need to gather, practice, rehearse your communication skills, and take action. Do your homework. Ask simple direct questions and look directly into your doctor's eyes when you ask. The most important question to ask is "Will this treatment or medication cause me to live longer or better?" Ask for the scientific evidence in support of any recommendation. The burden of proof lies with those selling the goods and services, not with the buyers. You need an acceptable level of proof before accepting your doctor's prescription.

I have a very dear friend who has severe arthritis. She was in a great deal of pain. I asked her to try a starch-centered diet for ten days. After ten days, I asked her how she was feeling. She said her pain went from an eight (on a scale of one to ten, ten being very painful) to a four! I was elated to see another success story. She continued on the dietary lifestyle change and continued to get better and better. Then she went to see her physician. Her physician immediately said that a starch-centered diet was not healthful, and he ordered a complete blood work. He came back and said that she must immediately start eating at least fish and eggs a couple times a week to protect her B12 levels, and she must eat yogurt at least twice a week for her calcium to protect her bones. As far as the vitamin B12 went, she could not have had a deficiency in ten days. In fact, there is no medical evidence of anyone developing this deficiency in ten months, or up to three years. Our bodies manufacture and recycle B12 bacteria, and we have storage for three or more years.

Ask your physician if they have ever had a patient suffering from any deficiencies come to see them? I am certain there is a plethora of patients who are suffering from abundances, however. The calcium? People in the countries with the highest milk consumption have the highest levels of hip fractures, and in the countries that have no dairy consumption, they have the strongest bones. I offered my friend the medical evidence of these studies to give her physician. However, she replied, "No, he is a doctor, and he knows more than I do." Oh, and my friend and her pain? It has gone back to crippling, and she is back on medications and regular visits to this doctor.

You will need to become a medical expert on your specific problems, and these days this is possible because of the Internet. Go to your search engine (Google, Yahoo) or a medical site like the National Library of Medicine (www.pubmed.gov). Do your homework before your doctor's office visit. My favorite place to go for research is (www.drmcdougall.com). This site has an incredible search engine for all medical articles written about everything you need to know to survive on a starch-centered diet.

When you are talking with your physician, you should hear from him or her, "Wow! You know as much about your diseases as I do." Your response should be, "Of course I do, doctor; these are my problems, and I want the best care and results possible." Let your physician know early in the appointment that you have done your homework. If you get a defensive reply, it is often because the physician is not up to speed on the current research. They are still operating as they did when they graduated from medical school, and they have not had the time to do more investigations. When you provide information, it may get in the way of their ego and cause you to hit a nerve!

Last night I had the opportunity to see a friend who had a heart attack recently and almost died. He told me the entire experience, which sounded quite frightening. His cholesterol was being managed with medications to bring it down to an acceptable level when he had his attack. He had major arteries that had been clogged, and they cleared them with angioplasty. I asked him what changes had he made since this occurred. He said that his doctor told him to stop smoking and to stop eating red meat. He said he has reduced his butter intake to a pound a month.

While visiting my friend, we were at a party where I watched him downing several pieces of a greasy cheese pizza, eating salami but passing on a piece of chocolate cake. "Because of my heart. Doctor's orders, guys. Sorry, can't eat the cake." What I find sad about this is that my friend is going to die. I wish his death certificate could say, "Cause of death: bad nutritional advice from his physician."

In some cases, I believe physicians are trying to get unhealthy wrecks to make *some* changes. They hand them all the information they can and hope they will educate themselves. Reality is, these people don't care and don't want to take time to extend their lives. I say this as it is; it is not an out for the individual to blame the doctor. They got themselves into this, even with all the information available.

I do want to share a positive experience. My father was diagnosed with stage 4 cancer at the age of ninety-one. He was referred to an oncologist to start him on his course of treatment options, which included chemotherapy and/or radiation.

My mother and I waited with my father in the waiting room. This was my first time in an oncologist's office. The air was thick with tension, as we all knew that everyone was dealing with the "big C." My father's name was called, and we were all invited in to join in him the examining room. The doctor came in, read the chart, and then sat down to talk to my father. He began with asking him about his practice in Texas, and then he asked, "Doctor, do you mind if I make some drawings and explain more about cancer to your family?" The doctor made drawings and explained each stage of cancer, where he was, and what was to be gained from treatment.

The doctor then pulled his chair close to my parents, and he looked them in the eye and said, "Doctor, the treatment would be worse than the cancer." He went on to say, "Ya know, Doc, from listening to you, you have a wonderful and rich life! How many more dinners out do you need, or how many more experiences do you need, to be able to say you've had a rich and fulfilling life?"

My mother started to cry, and the doctor immediately took her hand in his and said, "You have had a wonderful life together. I think it is best to just live this life and enjoy the time you have together, rather than make your husband sick and in pain from the treatment." I was so incredibly impressed with this doctor's manner and the respect he gave my parents.

My father had a different perspective on life since that appointment, and he was doing just what the doctored ordered. He was enjoying life. One morning about two months after this appointment, my father came into the kitchen and said, "WOW, I slept all night, and I have not done that in ten years! I feel fantastic." I offered to make him breakfast, and he asked for toast. We were talking about who I saw when I took the dog out. While I had the bread in the toaster, I heard what I describe to be a snore. When I looked over, my father was slumped in the chair. The medics arrived immediately, and he was pronounced deceased. My father could have had an agonizing, chemo-filled few more days, but instead he was able to make a choice and live life. Some physicians would have seen an opportunity to increase their billable time with treatment, but this physician chose to give educated options to his patient.

Sometimes greed can cause a physician to make bad decisions. In the same year as my father, my sister was rushed to the ICU because her lungs both failed. She was a smoker. She was in the ICU on assisted breathing and unresponsive. An intern came in and explained that she was on 100 percent oxygen and that normal atmospheric air is 20 percent. The amount of oxygen that she is breathing is destroying her lungs. He added, "I have worked here long enough to tell you that what you see will not get any better."

As a family, we knew we needed to have the machines turned off, but oh no, the physician had not made this determination. The physician came in and said, "We are going to put in a trach tube and then see how she is doing in a week." I mentioned that she had been in ICU on a breathing machine for a week, unresponsive on 100 percent O2. "Just how is adding a trach going to change the situation?" I asked. I got the normal response: "Are *you* a physician?" My mother, of course holding on to any hope, asked the physician, "Will this save her life?" and he replied, "We don't know. Let's just try it for a week."

After several phone calls, we were finally able to make the decision based on the information that we knew. Her lungs were destroyed, and she was not going to get better. We had the breathing tubes removed and remained by her side, and she rather quickly crossed over. The bottom line was that the physician could keep that patient for another week, generating more revenue for the hospital, knowing very well that her situation was not going to improve.

So if a starch-centered diet clearly shows improvement in disease, why are not more physicians vocal about this? If a physician were to suggest to a cancer patient to change his nutrition intake for treatment, I can guarantee you that they would be reported to the authorities or be permanently labeled as quacks or charlatans. A couple of doctors who have gone out on a limb have paved the way for others. It is a matter of time before doctors will be more accepting. Current treatment for cancer is not effective for most cancers. Ask a cancer nurse how many patients were helped by chemo and how many died from chemo. The science does not support traditional treatments for most cancers. We have also not made strides forward on most cancers—a few, yes, but the majority, no.

Another issue a physician faces is running a business. When a patient comes in to see their doctor, they want answers and to leave with a cure. If a physician suggested a change in lifestyle and diet, the patient would go around the corner to a physician who would gladly give them a prescription of drugs and tell them to go about their lives as normal.

Doctors are people, and they make mistakes. Do your own research, ask questions, and most important, ask for the scientific research to back up a procedure, and ask how this will improve your health. Don't be intimidated. If you ever feel you are intimidated, take your business someplace else. Don't be passive with your health and your body.

SURGERY

Almost every fat person has considered weight loss surgery. It appears to be the best option, a quick fix, and I will be forced to eat better, because I can't do it myself. Famous people are doing it all the time. It isn't my fault; it is genetic, and I need medical intervention.

Sounds great, but the truth is that they are not all success-ful. You can gain weight again even after the surgery. Surgery never fixes the root problem that caused the weight gain. Many physicians will make the claim that after surgery many co-morbidities are eliminated, and that it cures type 2 diabetes or sleep apnea. You will die if you don't do something about your weight. You have to be morbidly obese to get the surgery and that is based on your BMI (body mass index), a calculation of weight and height. Irony is, you have to lose a certain amount of weight before you have the surgery. This is protocol, and the intention is to demonstrate you can lose weight. If you can do that, why have invasive, expensive surgery? You can make the same claims for those who go on a starch-centered diet. A starch-centered diet is very cost effective, especially when you compare it to the cost of surgery.

What about the recover? You still have to change your diet with the bypass surgery but most of the time you can't eat the foods that make you healthy like complex starches! The more you mess with nature, the more problems you create. Ask any-one with gastric bypass surgery about their hair and protein and supplements; they no longer absorb the nutrients the same way as they did before. Ask about how they deal with their social life after surgery. I have a friend who had the surgery, and when he was asked if he would do it again, he said without hesitation, "Absolutely not." The only foods that do not make him throw up are the foods that caused his weight gain in the first place. Chocolate candy bars heated on the stove with heavy cream for a dessert soup is one food that does not hurt his "new" stomach or make him throw up. He still battles his weight; however, he cannot enjoy many of the great fiber-rich foods that could cause weight loss because of this surgery. Ask about dumping syndrome that occurs with gastric bypass. Fact is, you have to eat differently after the surgical intervention of weight loss surgery, so why not do it before? The overeating and obesity are symptoms of other issues in your life. If you cannot overeat, that addiction will be replaced by a different addiction. Many people turn to spending money, gambling, shopping, drinking, or sex as a means to get their fix.

There is a popular TV show currently that shows patients struggling with weight loss, and their surgery to correct it. I applaud the show for showing the failures as well as the successes. What is painfully evident is that they never really deal with the true *reason* they are obese. The doctors just cut their stomachs and tell them to eat less. The patients still struggle and deal with their original food issues. There was one episode in which after her surgery, the patient's husband, while driving her home from the hospital, drove her to a drive-through to get fast food. Why? Because she loved fast food, and he wanted her to have anything she wanted to be happy. It was like taking someone to dry out for alcohol addiction in a live-in treatment facility, and then to celebrate, taking them to a bar when they are released.

I am sure some people will claim that they could not lose weight without the surgery. It just baffles me why someone would take this step as opposed to going back to the basics of nature and eating a starch-centered diet and reaping the benefits of health and a slender body.

MEDICAL EQUIPMENT AND DEVICES FOR WEIGHT LOSS

This chapter could be summed up: "They don't work." We have all tried them. They were just another means to try to suck the money out of our wallets. I have had radio signals blasted into my fat. I have had platforms that I stood on that shook me until I felt like I was going to lose a filling. I have had high colonics, I have had my ass smeared with ox bile, clay, and electrodes to shock the fat away. You name it, I have tried it, and the only thing I lost was money. I think it is amazing how much money we will spend looking for hope. I am the first one to admit that I wanted to try it all in hopes of finding that magic bullet. The only magic bullet I found was through a starch-centered diet.

ANTIPERSPIRANT AND DEODORANT

OK, so why is this in here? Let me start with this: the larger you become, the more you start to smell. Part of the reason is because of the areas where bacteria can hide and grow. Most fat people are fastidious in keeping clean and odor-free. I used to use nuclear-powered deodorant. I remember telling my parents at a young age that I smelled. They didn't believe me, because I had not yet even started puberty. I finally lifted my arm and said, "Smell." They recoiled, ran to the bathroom, and handed me a can of deodorant. Part of the reason for body odor is from the sulfur in our diets. Meat has lots of sulfur. I used to sweat profusely, and my sweat was acidic. My sweat actually could remove the color from the lining of my clothes and eat through material, and it was toxic. I used to shower twice a day and lather on the deodorant.

Since being on a starch-based diet, I have been able to switch to deodorant and no longer use an aluminum-based antiperspirant. There are many articles linking Alzheimer's disease and aluminum. The most important piece of this topic is that once you eliminate the sulfur-producing products in your diet, you don't smell. I have heard this from others as well. I do not sweat profusely anymore, except at the gym.

SEX (FROM A MALE PERSPECTIVE)

You have to have something about sex in a book, or it will never sell. In all honesty, I want to share one benefit of a starch-centered diet. Now that you have a slimmer body and newfound energy, let's use it!

I first started this venture because I was tired of the side effects of blood pressure medications. Blood-pressure medications indeed reduce the pressure, and at times, we need that pressure. In simple terms, I had a flat tire. My local physician offered erectile dysfunction drugs like Viagra and Cialis. OK, I admit I tried them. At first, I was like, WOW! Reminded me of my youth. I had a side effect, however, that very few people experience, but it was frightening. Blood. I discussed this earlier and will spare the gory details again, but it was not pleasant.

One of the first indications of clogged arteries is mild erectile dysfunction. The vein that delivers blood to the penis is about the size of a small stir straw for coffee. Even if you do not suffer from ED (erectile dysfunction) you may notice that after a very fat-laden meal, you are not able to achieve a strong erection. This can be due to clogged arteries, but let's look at the mechanics of blood and fat also. Blood cells are flexible and pliable so that they are able to travel freely through the bodies inside every small artery. After a fatty meal, fat is attached to these cells, making them less flexible. They may have difficulty entering the small vein that makes a man's erection. Ever wonder why the erectile dysfunction medications all state not to take them with a fatty meal? Now you know.

Many people report stronger and better erections and new-found sex drive with a starch-centered diet. I can report that my libido has increased quite a bit. I do not take any pills or supplements for this. I would say after the first thirty days, I saw a change in erections and desire (my partner noted the changes as well). Aside from all the medical information and documentations of how a starch-centered diet can put lead in your pencil, let's look at the practical side. You have more energy, you are losing weight, and you don't have the aches and pains that you used to have. You are in better health, and you are starting to feel good about yourself. So have some fun. Take off your underwear, toss them at your partner, and run, scream-ing. "Catch me, catch me!"

VITAMINS AND SUPPLEMENTS

Eating a starch-based diet will provide you with all the nutri-ents you need, with the exception of vitamin B12. Our body stores vitamin B12, and we have stores in our body for years. It is recommended that anyone on a nonmeat diet supplement with vitamin B12. So where does vitamin B12 come from? It is bacteria that is excreted through poop. Animals eat it and ab-sorb the vitamin B12, and then people eat the animal to get the vitamin. In the old days, when manure was used as fertilizer, the vegetables were pulled from the ground, shaken off, and eaten. With today's sanitation standards, we wash away any residual vitamin B12. There are a few natural sources, but as a precau-tion, I personally take a small amount of vitamin B12 once a week. You can also have your vitamin B12 levels checked by a doctor with a blood test.

Vitamin D, which is not really a vitamin but rather a hor-mone, is one that has numerous benefits. If you are told you have low vitamin D levels, you should be told to go outside for fifteen minutes a day. Supplementation in studies was used as a last resort for a study group of institutionalized women, and it showed some success. Toxicity of over supplementation is much more of a risk. So if you are concerned, go outside in the sun!

As far as all the other vitamins and minerals are concerned, you could waste your money or look at a few facts. Minerals come from the soil, and the plants absorb them. Plants synthe-size vitamins, so when we eat plants, we obtain all the necessary vitamins and minerals we need. Some of you may think you need more. Have you ever considered what happens when you take too many? Every consider vitamin toxicity? Ever look at the data saying that supplementation can do more harm than help? Here is the scientific data. https://www.drmcdougall.com/health/education/health-science/hot-topics/nutrition-topics/supplements/.

If you want to be sure you are getting all the vitamins and minerals you need, besides a supplementation of vitamin B12, eat a varied diet of green and yellow vegetables and starches and spend some time outside. You are good to go!

I can burn a thousand calories in just twenty-five minutes. Just set the oven on high broil, toss in a pizza, and watch that baby burn.

Yes, I know some of you hate this word. I did, too. However, you will find that your body is going to start telling you to move. You do need to exercise in some form for a variety of reasons, but one of the most important for me is hunger control. Yep, exercise can actually help you manager your hunger. Also, it is going to help with sleep (which is very important), circulation, blood pressure, digestion, blood sugar, triglycerides, and more. Changing your diet is level one, and adding exercise bumps it up to the next level.

I found that an activity tracker helped me a great deal. I didn't realize just how sedentary I was until I got this gadget. It gives me motivation to get up and move when I have been sitting too long, and it also can give the awareness of how much one has done nothing but look at Facebook all day.

Remember that I said I was an all-or-nothing kind of guy? With exercise, this would be the way you could really burn out. Start small. Go for a walk. Later, maybe jog a little. Try walking faster each time. Do something. Get up and move. Walk around the block. Later, walk around the block twice. Wear your activity tracker and walk around a local mall. Get together a group of friends to walk with you. Love to swim? Go to the local pool. Join a gym and go.

Personal Trainer: Have you ever thought about using a personal trainer but felt uncomfortable or felt that you did not have the physical ability to utilize them? That was how I felt.

When I went to the gym, which was (and still is) always intimidating for me, I would watch the trainers working with clients and think, *Wow, I wish I could have a session. Once I am fit enough, I will.* My concern was that if I paid for a session, would I get some benefit from it? I really was still trying to figure out how everything worked in the gym.

I started going to the local gym and felt that I needed to do cardio. Reason was that I assumed people would look at my fat ass and say, "He really should be burning on cardio instead of pushing on the machines. Well, actually, he should be pushing his cheese and meat platter away."

I started with twenty minutes of cardio and then pushed on some of the machines. Later I got more and more confident on the cardio machines. Elliptical trainer was my favorite. I could watch TV and it was like running in sand and didn't hurt my joints. I got to where I was doing cardio for an hour and fifteen minutes and then twenty minutes of weight training. I made it a point to go to the gym three to four times per week. Gym staff members always came to ask how I was doing and if I had any questions.

I continued on the treadmill or elliptical, and to be honest, I felt great but didn't see any changes with my body. I would do sit-ups and everything else I could think of but was not really getting good results. I concluded that it was my age. I should not expect a younger-looking body, as I am approaching sixty, and that at this point I should just accept my lumps and bumps and continue eating healthfully.

I decided that rather than just give up, maybe I could try a couple of personal training sessions and get a few pointers or ideas to help my regular routine. When I went to the front desk to ask about making an appointment, I was surprised at the reaction. The trainer said, "Thank God!" I asked why the reaction. The trainer explained that he had watched me working out so hard and that with a few adjustments, we could fine-tune and get better results.

The first day I met Francisco, or Fran, my trainer, he reviewed my goals, what I wanted to achieve and repeated back to me what I wanted to accomplish to be sure we were to achieve *my* goals and not Fran's. A complete assessment was made, and we determined a plan that would work. The first thing that really impressed me was the time. My training session was going to be reduced to one hour, instead of my regular two hours! Fran explained that you can exercise with efficiency and gain great benefits. First, he explained, we needed to create a solid base—the core.

Core: At first I was a bit perplexed by the amount of time you should devote to developing your core. I wanted to lift heavy weights and make grunting noises the first day. I had no idea how important it was to strengthen your core for exercising better and achieving goals. He explained that not having a good core was like firing a cannon from a canoe. We knew how that would end!

You need a strong core base to work out without hurting yourself. Today when we work out with weights, Fran will remind me to use my entire core, not just my arms. My abs are used, my legs, my total body core is used when lifting a weight on a machine. This also prevents any injury.

Abdominal: Of course, I thought he would give me a bunch of crunches from hell. I have a lot of fat in that area, and I thought that was the only way to lose…nope! I was taught to use my core while I exercised, resulting in an incredible way to exercise your abs. Those are the planks.

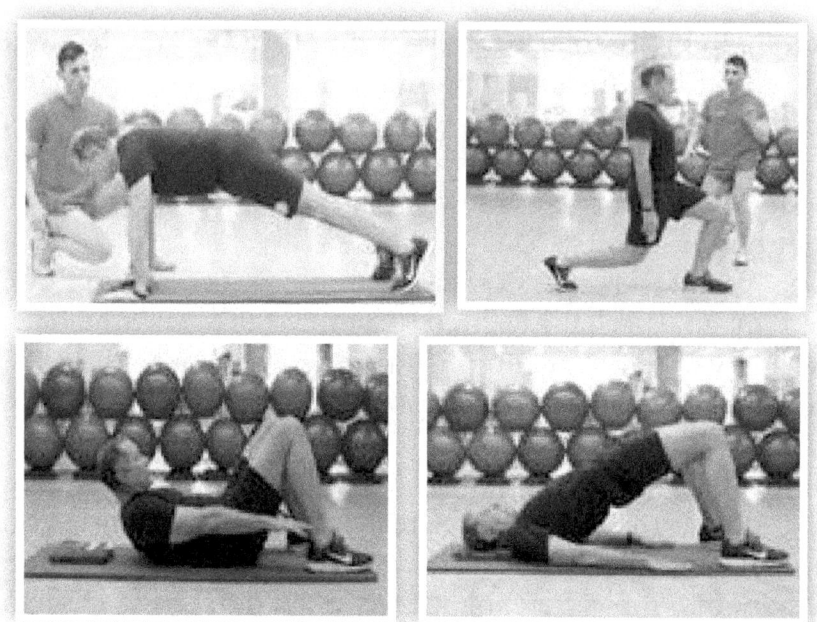

Planks, lunges, crunches, and bridges are excellent core-building exercises that can be done without a gym. A trainer can assure that you are doing these with proper form to prevent injury.

I was also surprised by the importance that was given to prevent injuries. Great pains were taken to be sure that nothing hurt me or provoked injury. I was impressed that most of the work we did together did not involve heavy weights but rather utilizing my body weight.

I have a bad habit of starting conversations when I'm tired so I don't have to keep exercising. Still, Fran was patient with me in this regard and would say, "Let's go" to proceed. I really surprised by his level of knowledge. Fran is not just a fit trainer, but he has a master's degree in fitness. He is well versed in the physiological and kinetic body functions but also in nutrition. It is important that even your trainer supports your starch-centered diet. Some trainers are still operating on the old paradigm that only flesh will build muscle.

I'll be honest with you, there were (and still are) days when I went to the gym, and I did not give 100 percent of myself. I can honestly say that there has not been a single session in which Fran has not devoted all his attention exclusively to me.

So you'll probably be wondering: Did you get the results you intended? The simple answer is yes. I also have a solid base so when I am traveling I can utilize the basics Fran gave me. Even if you only schedule a few sessions with a trainer, I encourage you to do so. Find a good trainer and go for a few sessions. See how form and function really change the impact of your workout. It isn't about lifting heavy things; it is about being fit, coordinated, and strong, and having a little guidance in achieving this is beneficial.

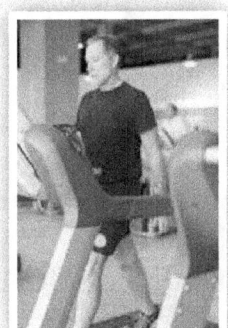
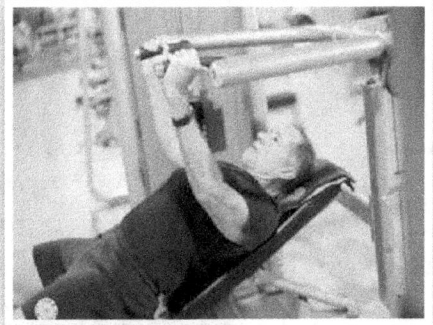
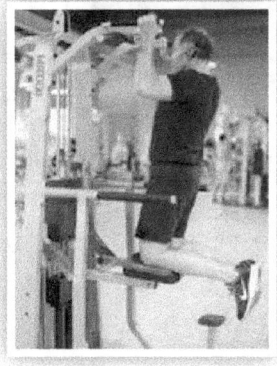

RESTAURANTS

I would have to say this is one of the biggest hurdles yet also the easiest to fix. Everyone at first thinks that they will just go to a vegan restaurant, and everything will be made to order and be perfect, since they don't eat anything that poops. The common problem you will face in vegan restaurants, as with most, is *oil*. Whenever someone contacts me and says their progress has completely stopped and that they have gained a little, I always ask, "How often have you gone out to eat?" This usually answers the question of the weight gain. Remember the oil you eat is the oil you wear.

How do we approach a restaurant? If I am invited as a guest to go to a particular restaurant, I will phone ahead a day or two before and speak with the chef. Ninety-nine percent of the time, they are more than willing to accommodate. Italian restaurants, unless they make their own pasta, have egg-free pasta. Most will have a marinara sauce that is oil-free and meat-free. You always can get a salad without cheese with some balsamic vinegar. Italian bread is usually wheat, water, salt, and yeast, so it's safe to eat. Mexican restaurants often have whole beans without meat products. Rice, beans, and a corn tortilla, and you are good to go. Japanese is easy—miso soup, udon noodle soup in vegetable broth, etc. Believe it or not, the easiest place is a steak house! You can get a plain baked potato and salad. The fancier the restaurant, the more willing they are to accommodate you, especially if you take the time to explain in advance.

You may be wondering why the initial reaction at a restaurant is that they are uncomfortable. A big part of this is because they want you to be a happy, satisfied customer. They are not used to the idea of not having an animal product or oil on the food. They think that you will not be happy or satisfied if they prepare it the way you ask. Even if the flavors are not just right, but they prepared it well, gush with praises. You will see them smile. They want you to be a happy customer. Most important, return to the restaurant. There is a Thai restaurant here that does an excellent job, and I host a large table with all starch-centered, no-oil-added food, and the restaurant is delighted.

Yes, you will run into some restaurants who will tell you they have nothing for you. If they cannot even think of a fresh vegetable salad, I would suggest thanking them and hand the menu back. It isn't worth the fight. If I think that they could. and I would like to return, I'll work with them. Ask yourself, "Is the juice worth the squeeze?" In other words, is it worth the battle and time to explain?

When traveling, you usually do not have the option to develop a relationship with a local restaurant. I have found an app for my phone that is helpful for locating a vegan restaurant or a health food store nearby. I have used this app all over the world. You can often talk a vegan restaurant into making you a special meal without oil. The app is called Happy Cow http://www.happycow.net/.

Again, going to a restaurant does not have to be a daunting experience. Call ahead and plan, and none will be the wiser. If you are unsure, always have something at home you can eat in an emergency, and perhaps eat something before you go out so you are not tempted. I have seen people fall off the program by going to a restaurant and declaring that there is nothing they can do, so they'll go ahead this once. It doesn't work. *Just say no.*

FEAST DAYS

There is a time to party and feast. These are special occasions. In the old days, people had a simple diet, and then on a special holiday, celebration, or religious observation, they would create a large feast. Royalty began eating these feast foods daily and they began suffering from the ailments that we do today. You can see the first clinical study, unofficially, in the Bible. In the book of Daniel (1:12–16), it says, "Please test your servants for ten days: Give us nothing but vegetables to eat and water to drink. Then compare our appearance with that of the young men who eat the royal food, and treat your servants in accordance with what you see." So he agreed to this and tested them for ten days. At the end of the ten days they looked healthier and better nourished than any of the young men who ate the royal food. So the guard took away their choice food and the wine they were to drink and gave them vegetables instead (NIV Bible).

Now days we have feast meals every day. Breakfast is Easter, with eggs and ham; lunch is Thanksgiving turkey and trimmings; dinner is Christmas, with a roast; and dessert is a birthday party, complete with cake and ice cream.

You remember the popularity about the book that claimed Europeans don't get fat. Here is the scoop. In general, Europeans go out for special occasions, not every day. In America, it is not unusual for someone to go out for at least one meal per day. Remember, the restaurants are going to use every ingredient to get you to come back. You all have experienced this when you travel. Most people claim the weight gain is from not exercising, but the truth is, it's from eating out all the time.

There are rich plant-based foods that should be eaten on special occasions. I will confess that at least once a week I have to make some melty cheese sauce, which contains a quarter cup of raw cashews. This is something I have for a special Friday night meal, for example. I might make guacamole with avocados for a special feast day. Not every day. A pie made with a crust of dates and walnuts—again, on a special evening, not every day. I can stop all progress with feast foods. You can gain weight with feast foods. Again, these are for special occasions; they are not something for every day!

Today I eat a very simple diet. Breakfast is oatmeal or cereal with oat milk; lunch is leftovers or a sandwich made with mashed spicy garbanzo beans, lettuce, and tomato, or a Caesar salad; and dinner it's rice and beans, a vegetable stew over rice, or whole-wheat couscous. There are special occasions when I have a feast. This could be a big bowl of chili with homemade tofu sour cream (low fat, not the commercial kind that is laden with fat) on a bed of rice served with melty cheese sauce, topped with some cubed avocado, and served with baked corn tortilla chips to dip into this luxurious concoction. This is not an everyday kind of meal. Yes, all the ingredients are on the approved list, but they are higher in fat. The scale and my pants can see a difference when I am eating feast foods more often than I should. Then I just go back to rice, beans, and a salad. This is all very satisfying. Remember, I do not measure portions. I eat what I want, whenever I want.

FLIGHT ATTENDANTS

It does not have to be stressful to maintain a starch-centered diet when traveling. I call the airlines ahead and ask for a vegan meal or a strict vegetarian meal. Just so you know, these items are not exactly healthful, but they are better than nothing. You will be given a pat of margarine that you should *not* eat. Usually the meal is a grain with sautéed vegetables (in oil, sigh), a fruit cup, and a salad. In my carry-on, I usually have allowable snacks or a piece of fruit. Be sure to bring some type of documentation that you require a special meal. It should be on your boarding pass. The reason I suggest this is that my special meal has been given to another passenger who decided to be healthy last minute and asked the attendant for a vegetarian meal. Attendants are quick to blame *you* for not ordering in advance. On an overseas flight, the attendant told me that I must have cancelled my meal because there wasn't any record. I was able to show on my boarding pass that was not the case. The flight attendant then brought me bread, fruit, and a salad but added, "Enjoy, this was *our* employee meal." If I had not provided any documentation, I would have been provided absolutely nothing.

When you have preordered your meal, and they are distributing bread, often the attendant will pass you by. You need to stop them and ask for egg-free bread. Ninety percent of the time I am told, "We have no gluten-free products." For some reason, people think that vegans are gluten intolerant.

The problem is that so many people claiming they can't eat gluten is that they are gluten ignorant. Yes, 1 percent of the population has a serious condition called celiac disease. True celiac people cannot tolerate gluten, and it can result in vomiting and other symptoms. There is a test for certain antibodies. Often celiac disease is mistaken for other problems, such as food intolerance or irritable bowel syndrome. Often people who have recently read a book about the terrible effects of grain on the body declare themselves gluten intolerant. This just adds confusion to others.

Preplan your travel. Call ahead to your destination. Call the cruise line. Call the hotel. Call the airline. Help them help you. Explain how simple it can be. Steamed vegetables and rice, plain baked potato and salad, etc. They want you to be happy.

BODY IMAGE

Growing up dealing with weight issues and fighting obesity affects how we see ourselves on a daily basis. I wake up every morning thinking about my weight, and I go to bed thinking about my weight. It took me a year to get rid of my "fat clothes." A day does not go by when I don't wonder if this all will end, and I will wake up in a fat body again, or the weight creeps back up. It has been three years, and my fears have not been realized. When I look into a mirror, my eyes do not see progress first, they see the flaws first. Reminds me of when you repaint an entire room, and it looks stunning. However, when you enter the room, your eye immediately goes to a flaw.

Changing your body image takes time. I have tried all the affirmations and standing in front of a mirror and saying all the magical words, but it happens slowly. I used to have great stress over wearing a bathing suit. I still am not comfortable. I would put on the bathing suit and then get a mirror and look to see just how much fat was oozing from the top. I didn't have a "muffin top," I had a "muffin toxic-spill explosion." I was also one of those kids who wore a T-shirt in the pool, thinking that it would hid my fat. After three years of weight loss, I am just now starting to be comfortable to walk around my house without a shirt on. True confession: I was petrified when I realized the photographer was going to take a picture of me without a shirt on. All the fears and negativity cropped up.

My trainer, Fran, shared that we have to realize that each one of us is different, and we each have a different type of body. I would show Fran a photo, and I would tell him, "I want to look like this." And he would affirm, "So do I, Christopher, but I will never be able to." Fran pushes me to learn to make the most of what I have and be happy with that. I will never be perfect in my eyes, but I am learning to be happy and proud of what I have accomplished.

Take photos of yourself in a mirror periodically. It is good to see the changes as they occur. It also helps to look at the pictures later to see yourself from a different perspective. I recently saw a photo of myself taken a year ago, and I thought, *I would not think that person looked fat at the beach*. This was a huge accomplishment!

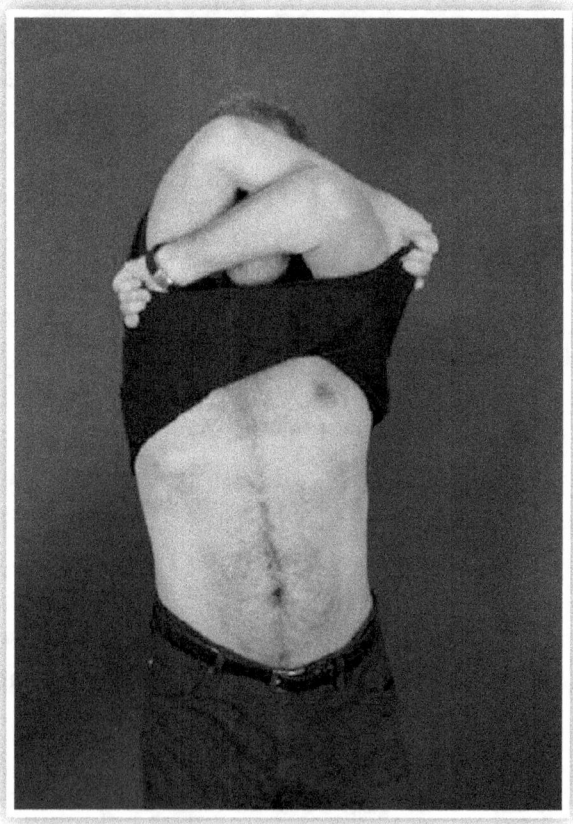

Going To "Mecca"

After I completed two years of a starch-centered diet, I decided to go the headquarters and see for myself the ten-day live-in program in Santa Rosa. I contacted Dr. McDougall to explain that I had already completed two years on the diet. Was it really worth it for me? Would I be bored attending this program? He assured me that many others had attended and felt it was well worth it, even though they had been on a starch-centered diet for a few years. We decided to go and find out for ourselves.

When we arrived we were pleasantly surprised at the hotel. Great accommodations with every imaginable facility you would want or expect. When we arrived, we were greeted by the McDougall staff who had our materials, room keys, schedules, etc. We were given a map to find our room. As we approached the entrance to the wing where our accommodations were located, an older woman ran up to me and asked, "Are you an artichoke or a broccoli?" I was somewhat perplexed and wondered if there was a mental health convention at this same hotel. I replied, "I am actually a cheese pizza." She politely smiled and said, "You won't be after *this* week."

We entered what I was expecting to be a normal hotel room, but instead we had a fantastic junior suite with a sofa, TV, desk, sitting area, huge comfortable beds. Everything was looking good! After a quick nap, we would go down for our orientation.

When arrived at the main meeting room, we were escorted to the room next door where there would be a few snacks. The table was spread with a feast of delights: hummus, vegetables, a huge variety of crackers, teas, water, coffee substitute, and plastic bags to make to-go packages. We were encouraged to eat as much as we wanted. The room was open 24-7. Also a table with medical information supporting what we were doing for the week.

In the opening the session we got to hear from John and Mary. At first I was not sure if it was John, because he was sporting a beard. Turns out they had just returned from Hawaii, and he grew it while on vacation and decided to keep it. He explained the week and what the expectations were. The biggest expectations were to be on time and to eat—to eat as much as we wanted, whenever we wanted, and not be hungry. I was loving this already. There would be lectures, escorted tours, exercise classes, yoga, and art, cooking demonstrations, restaurant outings, shopping, blood tests, doctor's visits, and more. It was a fully packed week but not overwhelming. Perfect balance. It was almost like a cruise ship without the movement.

Finally it was time for dinner. Three times a day, there was a luxurious spread of a variety of food all for the taking. You could return as many times as you wanted. There were to-go containers if you wanted to take some back to your room to put in the refrigerator or microwave in your suite. The food was really good, and it showcased the best of what a starch-centered diet can provide.

Forty-five people attended the week I was there. There were a couple others who had been on a starch-centered diet. The majority were there for medical reasons and desired a structured environment to see if they could get things under control without pharmaceutical intervention unless necessary. Dr. McDougall is a board-certified physician and can give prescriptions if needed. Some attendees were not sure if this was going to work for them, and some were hoping it would be what they needed. As each day passed, we could see changes and improvements in the unhealthiest. By the fourth day, you could see a change in the color of their skin. They were "pinking up." They had a healthy glow, and blood was filling vessels, making them look radiant.

On our final weigh-in and blood results, I got to witness the results and the impact of this week. There was one man who lost eleven pounds. Average weight loss was four pounds in ten days, eating all the food we wanted 24-7! People felt great. They looked great, and their blood results were astoundingly improved from when they arrived.

Some of you may ask, "Why do you call yourself a Starchiwhore?" According to the online Urban Dictionary, a "whore" of something is defined as someone who does something excessively. I eat a ton of starch now. I love starch. I am a whore for starch! At the McDougall clinic, I wore a shirt that said STARCHIVORE, and I told Dr. McDougall that I am officially a STARCHIwhore! He laughed and said, "Good luck on your new adventure, but with that name, I hope it isn't your last."

Was this trip worth it? Absolutely, and I would recommend it to anyone. The coordination that was required to make this week run as smoothly as it did was remarkable.

ADVANCED WEIGHT LOSS

This section really was not necessary for this book, but I wanted to share how I managed to shed the last bit of weight. I want to tell you that this is *not* the way one should eat a starch-centered diet. This is a "one-off." You will not feel good while on this diet. You *will* feel good on a regular starch-centered diet. This is a diet within a diet.

MARY'S MINIMCDOUGALL DIET

There is one minidiet that I do recommend that will give you results without much pain. In the early eighties, John and Mary

McDougall went on a diet of all potato and greens for ten days—just for the experience. They had hash browns for breakfast, baked potatoes and steamed frozen vegetables for lunch, and mashed potatoes with a salad for dinner. They both agreed that they were bored toward the end, but they each lost ten pounds, felt great, and continued their love for potatoes.

The principles are the same as with those of regular McDougall diet: it is starch-based with the addition of fruits and vegetables. The difference is that the goal is to lose weight quickly with as little effort as possible. This is just a temporary measure for a special occasion, not a lifestyle change. This is a temporary quick fix to be used as a tool for people overwhelmed by the initial challenges of starting on the McDougall program and/or to boost their progress when they feel that changes are coming too slowly. This is a nutritionally sound program that you, too, may want to follow.

Many people ask how they can dress their salads and what to put on top on their potatoes, etc. The idea is to create a bit of monotony. Eat simply, and if your food choices are a little boring during this minidiet, you will consume less and lose more.

Breakfast: Hash browns cooked on a dry skillet, no oil.
Lunch: baked potato and steamed frozen green and yellow vegetables
Dinner: mashed potatoes with a salad (lemon juice or vinegar for dressing) for dinner
Condiments: salsa, no-oil ketchup, no-oil barbecue sauce, vinegar

PRACTICAL APPLICATION OF "MARY'S MINIMCDOUGALL DIET"

Which starches are your favorites? Potatoes, sweet potatoes, winter squash, corn, beans, rice? Choose one or several to form the centerpiece of your diet. All of these can be found pre-cooked in packages in the frozen-food section of your grocery. Check the ingredients to make sure they are free of added fats, oils, or other harmful ingredients. The refrigerated section of the store will also have packages of fruits and vegetables for you to buy.

While root vegetables like potatoes and sweet potatoes provide well-rounded nutrition, grains and beans lack sufficient vitamins A and C to be eaten alone; therefore, add some fruit or green and yellow vegetables to make your grain and bean meals complete.

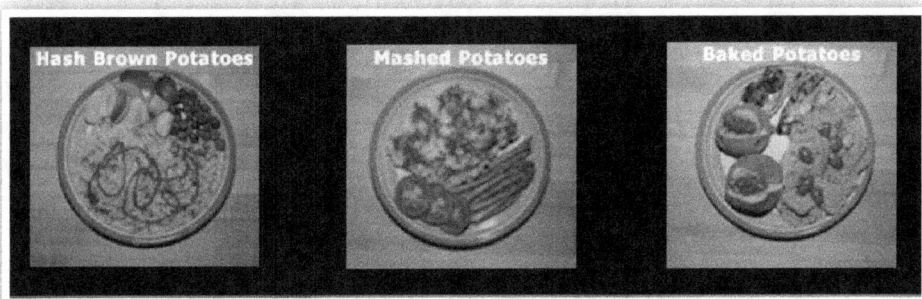

This is what Mary's Mini-Diet looks like day after day

I tried this minidiet, and it works well with minimal discomfort. The only negative aspect was the monotony; however, that was the point. If the food is less interesting, then we eat less, just enough to nourish our bodies. The weight loss was at a healthy rate, and I lost six pounds in one week. Muscle mass remained the same.

STARCHIVORE FAT BUSTER

This diet is thanks to a body builder who took the time to listen to what I wanted to accomplish and shed the last few pounds of body fat. The idea is to feed your body with complete nutrients constantly to trick your body into thinking that it is getting everything it needs so it can release the fat. It is almost like an intravenous nutrient supply. After you have done this for fourteen days, have a "cheat" day and then go back on the diet until you achieve your goal. April will use a similar plan while preparing for a competition. She is a professional body builder and will stay on this program for seventeen weeks. For meal six, April uses a protein drink. Because I avoid isolated proteins, it was suggested that I just add another meal. My plan is to try this for fourteen days only. Here is the modified plan:

- meal one: one cup raw oatmeal. Cook the oatmeal with as much water as you desire
- meal two: one cup cooked brown rice, one-quarter cup beans, and one cup raw spinach (no dressing or salt, just plain clean food)
- meal three: same as meal two
- meal four: same as meal two
- meal 5: same as meal two
- meal 6: same as meal two
- Drink plenty of water, a minimum of one liter and preferably two liters.

I decided to try this and keep a diary of my results.

Day one: WOW, there is so much food! I had no idea that by spacing my meals apart that I really can manage hunger so well. This is going to be a breeze.

Day two: OK, I think I can do this. I am not hungry, but I don't really feel satisfied. Maybe that is the point.

Day three: I have pain in my joints. I dreamed last night about melty cheese sauce and gravies made with raw cashews. I felt like I was catching a cold. I had diarrhea, which seems odd since I am eating mostly fiber. OK, this is *not* how I felt on the starch-centered diet at all. My body is demanding that I eat fat, because it does not like giving up the stored last bits of fat on my body. Went to the gym today and really could not have a good workout. I felt very weak. I am very grouchy and pretty much just want to be left alone. I am not enthusiastic about the food and just eat it to get it over with. From my previous diet experience, I know that day three is usually the worst. I will stick it out.

Day four: OK, this morning I have no pain, and I am starting to feel more "human." Had a pretty amazing textbook bowel movement, and things seem to be on track. Even from eating all this food, my stomach is flat. I am starting to get in a groove.

Day five: Feel OK, but not sleeping as long as I would like. Fewer dreams about cashews. Hunger has changed. It is no longer a "hankering" desire but rather urgency for the necessity of food. After I eat, I do not feel satiated, but I'm just not hungry. It is almost as if my body knows that it will receive nutrients but nothing more. I am dying to get on a scale to see if this is worth it. I purposely took the scale away so that I would not revert back to my old ways of weighing every day. Going to the gym again today and hopefully it will go better than day three. Back from the gym. Did not have a very good workout, and I am tired. Was not able to push myself as much.

Day six: Today I feel almost normal! Perfect, no, but normal. What I am finding is that my body tells me when I am hungry, but the pangs are minimal. Slept really well last night. Feeling more alert. The one item most noticeable is that my stomach is not as distended. I don't feel bloated at all. Another great bowel movement as well. Cravings have changed from cashews to veggie pizza and a glass of red wine. I am determined to stick with this through the fourteen days, and then I will have a starch-centered meal. My guess is that it will be mashed potatoes and mushroom gravy, which is my favorite!

Day seven: Nothing really remarkable to note. This may be TMI, but I had an incredible poop! Textbook perfect. No cravings, nothing much to report. I feel normal. I did run out of my home-cooked beans, so I bought canned. What an unpleasant difference. What do they do to canned beans to give you so much gas? I normally soak beans and put them in my InstaPot electric pressure cooker, and they are done in seventeen minutes. Still have not weighed but can tell a difference, and it is making me feel like I am losing body fat.

Day eight: Today went really well. Felt great and in a better mood. Bowel movements are textbook perfect. My body lets me know when I am hungry, and I eat. I am not as excited as I used to be about eating. It has become more of a function of necessity than desire.

Day nine: Feeling good. Stomach appears flatter, and clothes are looser in areas where they were not before. I am definitely losing fat. This is like "spot reduction" exercise, meaning that it will *not* take fat off a specific area, just like spot reduction exercise does not remove fat from the spot where you work it. Fat comes off based on where it landed. I think we all agree that love handles are the first place fat accumulates. Also, depending on the food you eat will determine where the fat settles. Have you ever encountered an alcoholic who has a trim body but a fat torso? My fat is all over the place. As a middle-aged man, it does accumulate around my stomach and love handles. Also my thighs. I have lost weight in my thighs and stomach but also can see it in my face. I am pretty sure this minidiet works, but again, I stress, it is *not* how a starch-centered diet should feel. A starch-centered diet is comfortable and not stressful or difficult at all. I have a few errands to run then take a walk. Tomorrow I have a big day at the gym.

Day ten: Today I feel really good. Sleeping well and have lots of energy, and I think today will be a good day. I ran out of spinach and had to substitute swiss chard. Love eating that raw. Tastes great.

Day eleven: Slept really well last night. Woke up and felt normal. Still do not have a clue how much weight or body fat I have lost. I feel really jazzed today and ready for my work-out session with my trainer. I have my meal packed, and I am ready to show that I can do this short-term diet and still work out as I normally do, and I will watch the pounds shed. Well, the workout was difficult. Not from what we normally do, but I just didn't have the energy that I normally do. My trainer asked me not to do the spin class but rather wait until I was off this minidiet and back to eating a starch-centered diet again. He can see that my energy levels are low. He did say that I look like I have lost weight in my face. I wanted to lose my love handles!

Day twelve: Same as yesterday, I am feeling pretty well. No real hunger, but at the precise moment that I am supposed to eat, BAM, I get hungry and have my meal, and then it is gone. What I have learned is that I still am in a habit of eating large portions three times a day. It is clear that small portions throughout the day are important, even on the regular starch-centered diet for those who want to lose weight and body fat. I am anxious to see what my body fat will be. Two more days to go.

Day thirteen: Really think I am used to this plan now. I am not real excited about food. It is more just something to do to get my nutrients. I am really missing the variety of food available on a starch-centered diet.

Day fourteen: This is it! Last day! The theory is that after today, I can have a cheat meal and then return to the plan. I decided to go ahead and weigh in for the results today and have my cheat meal tonight. Going with a group of friends to celebrate Chinese New Year. I already met with the restaurant and explained that I would like vegetables sautéed in water and rice.

Now, the drum roll...the results:

Beginning stats: weight 87.0 kilos (191.4 pounds), 24.2 percent fat

Ending stats: weight 84.3 kilos (185.46 pounds) 23.9 percent fat

So just about a six-pound weight loss in fourteen days. Fat percentage really didn't change much. I can see a difference in my body, and my clothes do fit differently. I kept all my muscle mass. It was a healthy weight-loss rate.

Ending assessment of this diet: not recommended. What I do recommend is eating a starch-centered diet and take advantage of the wonderful variety available to you. What I did learn from this minidiet was that eating small portions throughout the day is very important to prevent hunger, give your body a constant feed of nutrients. The monotony did prevent me from overeating. You can/could achieve the exact same results by following the basic starch-centered diet and space out your meals. On a starch-centered diet, I never felt low on energy, but on this minidiet I did. I was also in a horrible mood, and on the basic starch-centered diet, I was in a great mood and felt good.

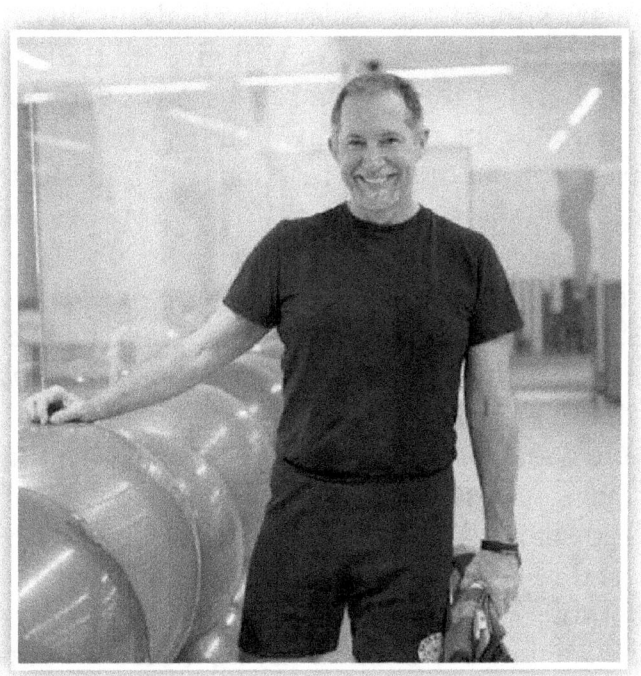

think all of you know that a properly planned plant-based diet—one that avoids all animal products, including meat, poultry, fish, eggs and dairy—is incredibly good for your health. Studies have shown plant-based eaters are thinner and have lower cholesterol and blood-pressure levels, a reduced risk of coronary heart disease and type 2 diabetes, and lower cancer rates—especially colorectal cancer.

Foods such as potatoes, rice, beans and lentils, nuts, whole grains, fruits, and vegetables offer a wealth of nutrients, fiber, and phytochemicals that have phenomenal health effects.

Starch-based vegan diets are higher in fiber, magnesium, folate, vitamins C and E, iron, and phytochemicals, while tending to be lower in calories, saturated fat, and cholesterol.

We know this inside, but we are bombarded with information that tells us the contrary and challenges us intellectually. Maybe you are still a little resistant to making this change, but if it were up to me, I would have you give up the fat-laden unhealthful food and embrace a starch-based vegan diet, not only for weight loss but for your individual health.

Here are a couple of other reasons why I advocate a starch-centered diet:

THE ENVIRONMENT

"Human health must be linked to planetary health, and how we feed ourselves has a major impact on the planet," says Dr. David Jenkins, – a Canada Research Chair in nutrition, metabolism and vascular biology, a professor in the department of nutritional sciences, faculty of medicine at the University of Toronto, and scientist at the Li Ka Shing Knowledge Institute of St. Michael's Hospital – became the first Canadian recipient of the Bloomberg Manulife Prize for the Promotion of Active Health. In a celebratory public conversation about his research, he shared with the crowd that he follows a vegan diet. It's the positive impact of plant-based eating on the environment, as well as animal welfare, that appeals.

Intensive animal agriculture is one of the leading sources of greenhouse-gas emissions and uses more water than any other human activity. Concentrated livestock operations can be major water polluters. Factory farms, as a whole, generate far more manure than can be properly disposed of. Nitrates, phosphates, bacteria, and viruses present in manure can seep into groundwater and pollute surface water, killing marine life and threatening public health.

According to Tony Weis, associate professor in the department of geography at the University of Western Ontario and author of *The Ecological Hoofprint: The Global Burden of Industrial Livestock*, increasing livestock production is a major force in the loss of biodiversity (the number of different species within an ecosystem), the pollution of waterways, and climate change.

Let's look at what will happen if we continue with the current trend. Within the past fifty years, increased consumption, urbanization, and population growth have increased worldwide demand for meat. Our appetite is voracious. It's predicted that by 2050, meat production will nearly double from what it is today. This enormous increase of meat and dairy consumption places great demands on the land, water, and resources needed for agriculture and the ensuing pollution burden. We are eating our planet to death!

ANIMAL WELFARE

Animals raised in intensive livestock operations are crammed together in pens or small cages or on feedlots, with minimal or no access to sunlight, fresh air, open pastures, or exercise, wading around in their own excrement, waiting to be killed. Many of us are unaware of the industrial methods—from farm to slaughterhouse—that put steak, chicken, pork, eggs, and milk on our table. My mother, who loves to eat meat, refuses watch any documentary that shows how the meat gets to her table. The documentary *Food, Inc.* I think will change your views.

For years, we've been making dietary decisions based on the calories, fat, fiber, cholesterol, or vitamins and minerals foods contain. There are, however, mounting concerns over freshwater supply, loss of biodiversity, and climate change. It's time to make the shift away from animal foods and toward a plant-based diet.

FOR YOU

It just makes sense. If you want to look great, feel great, and do something to save the plant, a starch-centered diet is the key, the magic bullet! What could be simpler? You eats lots of good food, as much as you want, you get healthier, help prevent cancers, diabetes, hypertension, heart disease, and a myriad of other diseases, and on top of all this, lose weight without a battle?

Remember, you may not be in the best health right now, but it isn't all your fault. It is the food